# Senseless Violence and Its Ramifications

The baby boomer generation grew up in the 1950s when there existed the general belief that the Cold War was the greatest threat to the world order, and a frightening possibility. It was difficult to believe, then, that it could get worse, but the same threat of violence is now a daily occurrence around the globe. People are being shot, slaughtered, maimed, and disappear for a multitude of reasons, none having any connection, most of the time, with the victims. The scale of loss when these tragedies occur is devastating, leaving the public as well as policy makers and legislators scrambling for solutions, clarification, and understanding of how we have become a society where violence is so rampant, so frequent, and so senseless. This book includes contributions by leading experts on violence and its ramifications, who review the devastation, reasons, and consequences of violence which is senseless, cruel, and aims to hurt and destroy anyone in its path.

This book was originally published as a special issue of *The Journal of Psychology*.

**Ami Rokach** is a clinical psychologist, specializing in addressing loneliness, anxiety, intimate and societal relationships, sexuality, and dying. He teaches Psychology at York University, Canada; the Centre for Academic Studies, Israel; and Walden University, USA. He is the Executive Editor of *The Journal of Psychology: Interdisciplinary and Applied*.

T0346601

# Senseless Violence and Its Ramifications

*Edited by*
Ami Rokach

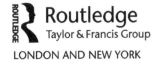

LONDON AND NEW YORK

First published 2018 by Routledge

2 Park Square, Milton Park, Abingdon, Oxfordshire OX14 4RN
52 Vanderbilt Avenue, New York, NY 10017

*Routledge is an imprint of the Taylor & Francis Group, an informa business*

First issued in paperback 2019

*British Library Cataloguing in Publication Data*
A catalogue record for this book is available from the British Library

ISBN 13: 978-1-138-09112-2 (hbk)
ISBN 13: 978-0-367-23429-4 (pbk)

Typeset in MinionPro
by diacriTech, Chennai

**Publisher's Note**
The publisher accepts responsibility for any inconsistencies that may have arisen
during the conversion of this book from journal articles to book chapters, namely
the possible inclusion of journal terminology.

**Disclaimer**
Every effort has been made to contact copyright holders for their permission to
reprint material in this book. The publishers would be grateful to hear from any
copyright holder who is not here acknowledged and will undertake to rectify any
errors or omissions in future editions of this book.

# Contents

*Citation Information*                                                                                      vii

*Notes on Contributors*                                                                                     ix

Senseless Violence: A Twenty-First Century Epidemic—An Introduction                        1
*Ami Rokach, with contribution by Karishma Patel*

1   Exploring the Interconnected Trauma of Personal, Social, and Structural
    Stressors: Making "Sense" of Senseless Violence                                                    5
    *Mona M. Abo-Zena*

2   In Search of Meaning: Are School Rampage Shootings Random and
    Senseless Violence?                                                                                   21
    *Eric Madfis*

3   A Case Study of Paternal Filicide-Suicide: Personality Disorder, Motives, and
    Victim Choice                                                                                         36
    *F. Declercq, R. Meganck, and K. Audenaert*

4   Violence is Rare in Autism: When It Does Occur, Is It Sometimes Extreme?             49
    *C. S. Allely, P. Wilson, H. Minnis, L. Thompson, E. Yaksic, and C. Gillberg*

5   Senseless Violence Against Central American Unaccompanied Minors:
    Historical Background and Call for Help                                                           69
    *Cheryl B. Sawyer and Judith Márquez*

6   Violent Video Games Exposed: A Blow by Blow Account of Senseless
    Violence in Games                                                                                     76
    *Andrew Krantz, Vipul Shukla, Michele Knox, and Karyssa Schrouder*

# CONTENTS

7  Making Sense of the Brutality of the Holocaust: Critical Themes and New
   Perspectives                                                          88
   *Eric D. Miller*

   Epilogue—Senseless Violence: An Overview                              107
   *Ami Rokach*

   *Index*                                                               113

# Citation Information

The chapters in this book were originally published in *The Journal of Psychology*, volume 151, issue 1 (January 2017). When citing this material, please use the original page numbering for each article, as follows:

**Chapter 1**
*Exploring the Interconnected Trauma of Personal, Social, and Structural Stressors: Making "Sense" of Senseless Violence*
Mona M. Abo-Zena
*The Journal of Psychology*, volume 151, issue 1 (2017) pp. 5–20

**Chapter 2**
*In Search of Meaning: Are School Rampage Shootings Random and Senseless Violence?*
Eric Madfis
*The Journal of Psychology*, volume 151, issue 1 (2017) pp. 21–35

**Chapter 3**
*A Case Study of Paternal Filicide-Suicide: Personality Disorder, Motives, and Victim Choice*
F. Declercq, R. Meganck, and K. Audenaert
*The Journal of Psychology*, volume 151, issue 1 (2017) pp. 36–48

**Chapter 4**
*Violence is Rare in Autism: When It Does Occur, Is It Sometimes Extreme?*
C. S. Allely, P. Wilson, H. Minnis, L. Thompson, E. Yaksic, and C. Gillberg
*The Journal of Psychology*, volume 151, issue 1 (2017) pp. 49–68

**Chapter 5**
*Senseless Violence Against Central American Unaccompanied Minors: Historical Background and Call for Help*
Cheryl B. Sawyer and Judith Márquez
*The Journal of Psychology*, volume 151, issue 1 (2017) pp. 69–75

**Chapter 6**
*Violent Video Games Exposed: A Blow by Blow Account of Senseless Violence in Games*
Andrew Krantz, Vipul Shukla, Michele Knox, and Karyssa Schrouder
*The Journal of Psychology*, volume 151, issue 1 (2017) pp. 76–87

## Chapter 7

*Making Sense of the Brutality of the Holocaust: Critical Themes and New Perspectives*
Eric D. Miller
*The Journal of Psychology*, volume 151, issue 1 (2017) pp. 88–106

## Epilogue

*Senseless Violence: An Overview*
Ami Rokach
*The Journal of Psychology*, volume 151, issue 1 (2017) pp. 107–111

For any permission-related enquiries please visit:
http://www.tandfonline.com/page/help/permissions

# Notes on Contributors

**Mona M. Abo-Zena** is a visiting assistant professor at Brown University, USA.

**C. Allely** is a lecturer in Psychology at the University of Salford in Manchester, UK, and is an affiliate member of the Gillberg Neuropsychiatry Centre at Gothenburg University, Sweden.

**K. Audenaert** holds an MD. He is a psychiatrist and professor at Ghent University, Belgium.

**F. Declercq** holds a PhD in clinical psychology. He is a professor at Ghent University, Belgium.

**C. Gillberg** is a professor of Child and Adolescent Psychiatry at the Gillberg Neuropsychiatry Centre, University of Gothenburg, Sweden, and the University of Glasgow, Scotland.

**Michele Knox** is a professor of Psychiatry and licensed clinical psychologist at College of Medicine, University of Toledo, USA.

**Andrew Krantz** recently received his BA in Psychology from the University of Toledo, USA. He plans to pursue graduate studies in clinical psychology, with research interests in adolescent and youth psychology.

**Eric Madfis** is an assistant professor of Criminal Justice at the University of Washington, USA, where his research focuses on theoretical criminology, the sociology of deviance, mass murder, hate crime, school shootings, and the school-to-prison pipeline.

**Judith Márquez** is a professor of Bilingual Education and English as a Second Language (ESL) at the University of Houston–Clear Lake (UHCL), USA.

**R. Meganck** holds a PhD in clinical psychology. She is a professor at Ghent University, Belgium.

**Eric D. Miller** is an associate professor of Psychology at Kent State University (East Liverpool Campus), USA.

**H. Minnis** is Professor of Child and Adolescent Psychiatry at the Institute of Health and Wellbeing, University of Glasgow, Scotland, and her research interests are maltreatment-associated psychiatric problems.

# NOTES ON CONTRIBUTORS

**Karishma Patel** is an undergraduate student in the Psychology Program at York University, USA, and will be graduating in 2017 with a BSc in Psychology. Her therapeutic and research interests include loneliness, palliative care, and neurological disorders.

**Ami Rokach** is a clinical psychologist, specializing in addressing loneliness, anxiety, intimate and societal relationships, sexuality, and dying. He teaches Psychology at York University, Canada; the Centre for Academic Studies, Israel; and Walden University, USA. He is the Executive Editor of the *Journal of Psychology: Interdisciplinary and Applied*.

**Cheryl Sawyer** is Assistant Professor at the School of Education, University of Houston–Clear Lake, USA.

**Karyssa Schrouder** is currently a second-year medical student at the University of Toledo College of Medicine and Life Sciences, USA.

**Vipul Shukla** is a graduate student in the LGBT Health Policy and Practice Program at George Washington University, USA.

**L. Thompson** is a research fellow at the Institute for Health and Wellbeing, University of Glasgow, Scotland.

**P. Wilson** is Professor of Primary Care and Rural Health in the Institute of Applied Health Sciences at the University of Aberdeen, Scotland.

**E. Yaksic** is the founder of the Serial Homicide Expertise and Information Sharing Collaborative, USA, co-founder of Northeastern University's Atypical Homicide Research Group, and a member of the Murder Accountability Project's board of directors.

# Senseless Violence: A Twenty-First-Century Epidemic—An Introduction

Ami Rokach

With contribution by Karishma Patel

Before the collapse of the Soviet Union we, in the Western Hemisphere, used to think that the Cold War, and threat of an all-out war, was the worst possible outcome of the hostilities between East and West. Now, in the second decade of the twenty-first century, we know that it can get worse, it may happen daily, and it may occur anywhere where there are people who can get hurt: young, old, innocent, and unaware of the reasons that they are targeted.

The scale of loss when these tragedies occur is devastating, leaving the public as well as policy makers and legislators scrambling for solutions, clarification, and understanding of how we have become a society where violence is so rampant, so frequent, and so senseless.

Following is a sample of such senseless violence that has occurred within the last 18 months.

1.  A recent report (Sanchez, Lister, Bixler, O'Key, Hogenmiller, & Tawfeeq, 2016) indicates that since its inception, ISIS (the Islamic caliphate that is dedicated to conquering the Western world and imposing the strictest Islamic rule) has carried out over 100 terrorist attacks in approximately 20 countries other than Iraq and Syria, which they initially targeted. Outside of those two countries, they have killed almost 1,280 people and injured more than 1,770 others. Some of the more commonly known and recent ISIS attacks include the two explosions at the Brussels airport on March 22, 2016, in which ISIS confirmed that its fighters had carried out the attack. Another example is the attack that occurred on March 19, 2016, in which a suicide bomber struck a busy tourist area in Istanbul, Turkey, and the minister declared that the attacker was definitely linked to ISIS. That attack alone injured 36 and killed four people. Since 2014, ISIS has expanded and is now wreaking havoc in many more countries than before. It is, now, more active in posting extremely torturous photos and video content.
2.  Thirty people were killed and 45 others wounded in a double suicide bombing attack in Damascus, Syria, on March 15, 2017. The first attack took place at the Justice Palace, the main judicial building. When security officers tried to arrest a man who was carrying grenades and a shotgun, he forced his way into the building and blew himself up, killing and injuring lawyers, judges, and innocent people visiting the palace. In the second suicide bombing attack, a man fleeing the authorities ran into a restaurant and detonated his explosive vest (Stanglin, 2017).
3.  In London, UK, a terror attack unfolded on a Wednesday afternoon during which a terrorist drove onto the pedestrian sidewalk on Westminster Bridge toward the Palace of Westminster before crashing into a railing. The terrorist ran into New Palace Yard

and stabbed a police officer multiple times before being shot and killed. His terror attack killed four people and injured around 20 others (Addley & Graham-Harrison, 2017).

4.  A crowded vegetable shopping market was the target of a terror attack in Parachinar, Pakistan, on January 21, 2017. A bomb planted in a vegetable crate exploded and killed 20 people while injuring 43 others. This attack was the first terrorist attack of the year for Pakistan with the Pakistani Taliban claiming responsibility (Masood & Khan, 2017).

5.  Thirteen people were left wounded in shootings across Chicago, and one man was pronounced dead on Thursday, July 21, 2016. Another shooting was done by a cop, after the man shot an officer in the leg in South Loop Park. Around 9:15 pm, a fatal shooting involving a 29-year-old man who was walking up the 6700 block of South Chappel occurred when he was shot in the chest by an unknown person. He was escorted to a Cook County hospital where he was pronounced dead (Armentrout, 2016).

6.  One of the most deadly shootings to ever occur in the United States left the city of Orlando in shock. The shooting occurred at a gay night club called Pulse. Occurring on June 12, 2016, 49 people were found to be dead and 53 others injured after the shooter attacked during nightclub hours. The attacker was identified as 29-year-old Omar Mateen. The gunman had taken several hostages that were found to be hiding in the stalls in the washrooms. The police were successful in taking down Mateen, after a supposed three-hour standoff. According to reports, Mateen has sworn allegiance to ISIL, and the FBI remains unsure and skeptical of reports claiming that Mateen was a regular at the gay nightclub and had used gay dating sites previously. Despite the claims, the CIA said it didn't find any strong links between ISIL and Mateen (Berman & Zapotosky, 2016).

7.  During a time of grievance and mourning, a bomb attack left many witnesses in Pakistan horrified. Around 100 Pakistani lawyers gathered at a government-run hospital in Quetta, Pakistan, on August 8, 2016. Lawyers had gathered at the Quetta Civil Hospital to express their condolences for their killed colleague, prominent attorney Bilal Kasi. At this gathering, a Taliban terrorist group known as Jamaat-ur-Ahrar targeted the group of lawyers with a planned suicide bomber attack, killing 70 people and wounding nearly 100. The motive behind the attack is still unclear, but it has been speculated by Ali Zafar, the president of the Supreme Court Bar Association of Pakistan, that lawyers are being targeted as they support democracy and people (Associated Press, 2016).

8.  A night of celebration in Nice, France, was quickly turned into a horrendous nightmare on July 14, 2016. Following a fireworks show in celebration of Bastille Day, a large 19-ton truck drove into the celebrating crowds. The driver, Mohamed Lahouaiej Bouhlel, drove the truck for approximately 2 km before finally being shot dead by police. His terror attack killed around 84 people, including 10 children (Chazan et al., 2016).

9.  The most surprising terror attacks are those that are conducted by co-workers and neighbors. Syed Rizwan Farook and Tashfeen Malik were a married couple that resided in San Bernardino, California, in the United States. They opened fire at a holiday party, specifically the party at Inland Regional Centre on December 2, 2015, where Syed Rizwan Farook had been employed for the last five years. It was speculated that they had plotted the terror attack in advance, before getting engaged. They killed 14 people and injured around 21 others before they were killed in an exchange of gunfire with police (Calamur, Koren, & Ford, 2015).

This book is dedicated to all those innocent victims who were targeted although they have done nothing to cause the violence that was directed at them. We hope that we will succeed in highlighting the psychological ramifications of senseless and unpredictable violence, and bring about researchers' and clinicians' interest in exploring, understanding, and formulating ways of reducing, if not eliminating, the suffering of those who have been so harmed with no fault of their own. I will briefly overview the articles that we included in this publication.

Abo-Zena's article opens this issue with an attempt to make sense of the senseless violence. The article defines senseless violence and then explores microaggression and violence that is politically and socially motivated. It concludes by suggesting ways that can be utilized to reduce that violence.

Madfis discusses the concepts of pointlessness, patternlessness, and deterioration of multiple-victim school shootings gleaned from empirical research about the phenomenon. The paper reviews the academic literature on school rampage shootings and explores the extent to which these attacks are and are not random acts of violence.

Declercq et al. address a specific and most disturbing case of senseless violence, that of a parent killing his/her child. As unfathomable as it is, we hear of such cases, in some cultures more frequently than in others. The paper presents a fully documented case of a paternal filicide, in which two motives were present: spousal revenge and altruism. The choice of the victim was in line with emerging evidence indicating that children with disabilities in general and with autism in particular are frequent victims of filicide-suicide. The father was diagnosed with a schizoid personality disorder.

Allely explores the research findings that point out the increased risk of violence meted on individuals with autism spectrum disorder (ASD), while the general public may believe that those autistic individuals are actually the perpetrators. There is, adds Allely, a small subgroup of individuals with ASD who do exhibit violent offending behaviors, and our previous work has suggested that other factors, such as adverse childhood experiences, might significantly contribute to their violent behavior. The author adds that school shootings and mass killings are not uncommonly carried out by individuals with neurodevelopmental disorders, a finding that requires further research and clarification.

Sawyer and Márquez shed light on the "collateral" sufferers of senseless violence that we hardly hear about. Addressing the situation on the southern border of the United States, they highlight what is experienced by the unaccompanied children from Honduras, Guatemala, and El Salvador who illegally cross the Mexican border into the United States. Many of these children leave home to flee violence, starvation, impoverished living conditions, or other life-threatening situations. They point out that the untreated traumatic events experienced by this population can develop into post-traumatic stress disorder, a potentially life-changing and physically threatening psychological and medical issue. There is an urgent need not only to allow those kids to enter the United States, but also to provide them with treatment of the acute stress, anxiety, and depression associated with traumatic events so that they can move forward with their lives.

Krantz' et al. article is exploring the connection between violent video games (that youngsters may find alluring) and desensitization to violence, decreased empathy and prosocial behavior, and aggressive thoughts and behaviors. The author alerts us to the fact that although research indicated that the connection does exist, these video games continue to be available and used widely, despite their negative influence on the players and indirect promotion of increased tolerance of violent behavior.

Miller examines the Holocaust, which he terms "one of history's greatest atrocities," and offers an analytic, integrative review of select themes associated with the Holocaust. Miller emphasizes the importance of having a greater understanding of the sheer brutality of violence perpetuated in the Holocaust. As part of this discussion, considerable attention is given to how Internet-based photographs and videos from the Holocaust era can provide greater insight into understanding the evil associated with this genocide.

## References

Addley, E., & Graham-Harrison, E. (2017, March 22). London attack: what we know so far. *The Guardian*. Retrieved from www.theguardian.com/uk-news/2017/mar/22/attack-houses-parliament-london -what-we-know-so-far

Armentrout, M. (2016, July 22). Cops: man shot dead on South Side. *Chicago Sun Times*. Retrieved from http://chicago.suntimes.com/news/cops-man-shot-dead-on-south-side/

Associated Press (2016, August 8). 'An attack on justice': 70 killed in hospital bombing in Pakistani city of Quetta. Retrieved August 9, 2016, from www.cbc.ca/news/world/pakistan-quetta-hospital-bombing-1.3711312

Berman, M., & Zapotosky, M. (2016, June 20). What we still don't know about the Orlando shooting rampage. *The Washington Post*. Retrieved June 20, 2016, from www.washingtonpost.com/news/post-nation/wp/2016/06/19/what-we-still-dont-know-about-the-orlando-shooting-rampage/?utm_term=.ff38a3569d93

Calamur, K., Koren, M., & Ford, M. (2015, December 3). A day after the San Bernardino shooting. *The Atlantic*. Retrieved August 12, 2016, from www.theatlantic.com/national/archive/2015/12/a-shooter-in-san-bernardino/418497/

Chazan, D., Willgress, L., Jalil, J., Morgan, T., Turner, C., Allen, P., ... Smith, S. (2016, July 17). Nice terror attack: 'soldier of Islam' Bouhlel 'took drugs and used dating sites to pick up men and women.' *The Telegraph*. Retrieved August 11, 2016, from www.telegraph.co.uk/news/2016/07/17/nice-terror-attack-police-vans-blocking-promenade-withdrawn-hour1/

Masood, S., & Khan, I. (2017, January 21). Pakistani Taliban claim deadly market bombing. *The New York Times*. Retrieved from www.nytimes.com/2017/01/21/world/asia/pakistani-taliban-claim-deadly-market-bombing-in-parachinar.html

Sanchez, R., Lister, T., Bixler, M., O'Key, S., Hogenmiller, M., & Tawfeeq, M. (2016, April 7). ISIS: 75 attacks. 20 countries, 1,280 killed. *CNN*. Retrieved April 11, 2016, from www.cnn.com/2015/12/17/world/mapping-isis-attacks-around-the-world/index.html

Stanglin, D. (2017, March 15). At least 30 killed in suicide bombings at Damascus justice building, cafe. *USA Today*. Retrieved from www.usatoday.com/story/news/2017/03/15/reports-suicide-bomb-kills-25-justice-ministry-damascus/99200378/

# Exploring the Interconnected Trauma of Personal, Social, and Structural Stressors: Making "Sense" of Senseless Violence

Mona M. Abo-Zena

**ABSTRACT**

Although violence is a timeless characteristic of human behavior and history, its prevalence and many forms are proliferated repeatedly through the media. In particular, "senseless" violence against both random and targeted victims puzzles and petrifies onlookers and survivors. Integrating developmental psychology with critical theory, this manuscript begins with a conceptual definition of senseless violence that is coupled with a mapping of the personal, social, and structural etiologies of such violence. This inquiry explores the origins, contexts, and varied manifestations of violence, helps redirect sense-making around such violence, and informs how to cope with and possibly reduce or mitigate it. Utilizing a person-centered perspective from multiple points of view, the analysis focuses primarily on the everyday or chronic experiences of stressors and their relation to internalized and externalized types of violence (i.e., mass shootings, interpersonal violence, self-injury). The manuscript concludes with ways to reduce violence and promote justice on personal, social, and structural levels.

*True peace is not merely the absence of tension; it is the presence of justice.*
    —*Dr. Martin Luther King Junior, 1958* (King, 1958/2010, p. 27)

Headlines around the world repeatedly force us to consider atrocities that affect both random and targeted victims (e.g., terrorist attacks, genocides). While many of us puzzle over the headlines of large-scale, heinous violent acts, individual atrocities of senseless violence are also proliferated (e.g., the killing of unarmed Black men and women while in police custody), and include the countless micro-aggressions and violent acts committed in interpersonal relationships. How can we broaden our conceptualization of senseless violence in order to better understand its personal, social, and structural connectedness so that we can reduce violence and promote justice within and throughout these relationships and systems? In particular, this article focuses on everyday interactions and experiences in order to re-center on bodies that produce and encounter violence in many forms.

This manuscript includes a conceptual re-definition of senseless violence and is coupled with a mapping of the personal, social, and structural etiologies of such violence. Understanding the origins and manifestations of violence facilitates making "sense" of otherwise pointless seeming behaviors, and informs how we may cope with and possibly reduce mal-adaptive emotions and behaviors. While we locate violence within broader socio-political-economic-historical contexts, the manuscript focuses primarily on the everyday or chronic experiences of stressors and their relation to internalized and externalized types of violence (e.g., mass shootings, interpersonal violence, and micro-aggressions that are race, gender, sexuality, class, or ability based), as well as the relation between victim and victimizer. Applying a critical, contextually grounded, developmental system theoretical lens allows for better understanding the interplay between victim and victimizer, which may reduce violence and promote justice on personal, social, and structural levels.

### Views on the Origins and Representation of Senseless Violence

Violence, like other forms of behavior, is socially mediated and individually experienced. Contemporary scholarly foci regarding violence often associate the role of media and "media hype" in widely broadcasting and replaying varied acts of "street" and "senseless" violence in the 24/7 hour news cycle (Crary, 2013, Vasterman, 2005). Analysis of gratuitous violence as well as its media representation highlights how the geography of fear has racist and sexist overtones that are structurally proliferated, as well as experienced personally and interpersonally (Aitken, 2001, Chiricos & Eschholz, 2002). This ongoing media cycle and re-presentation of violence and its alleged perpetrators has many variations, but violence itself has persisted historically throughout human society. Within the range of human emotion and behavior throughout history, violence is a universal form of behavior, but manifests in different ways in part due to cultural and contextual values surrounding its production and form (Block, 2000). Given this prevalence through human history, social scientists advocate shifting the focus from strictly condemning particular forms of violence to comprehensively understanding violence within its context (Aitken, 2001; Arendt, 1970; Block, 2000). In this light, violence can be both a creative and destructive force that has mostly been studied through anthropological, psychological, sociological, and historical lenses in order to explore the ways in which it is represented, rather than analyzing the circumstances surrounding violent behaviors and how they are experienced and understood at an individual level (Schmidt & Schröder, 2011).

For this reason, holistically defining and making sense of the phenomena of violence requires incorporating a psychological framework to understand how individuals' co-construct their behaviors, both their external observable action and internal thoughts, as influenced by a range of contextual factors over time (Li, 2003). A phenomenological theory of violence encompasses the physical, psychic, and structural manifestations of violence and explores them from the perspective of the person or subject (Staudigl, 2007). In contrast to aggression, violence is intended to produce extreme physical harm, such as injury or death (Bushman, Newman, Calvert, Downey, Dredze, Gottfredson, & Romer, 2016). Although "senseless" violence is considered particularly abhorrent, its representation is veiled by considerable subjectivity surrounding its definition. For example, "senseless" violence is often referenced as "random," "rampage," or "street" partly because of what is considered the inadequate cause or reason for the violence; meanwhile, there is evidence that 78% of school shooters were socially marginalized, suggesting that robust correlations that provide insights into systematic patterns do exist (Newman, Fox, Harding, & Mehta, 2004). We also know that despite the similar outcomes, "street" shootings (i.e., usually not perceived as "senseless") and "rampage" school shootings (i.e., widely perceived and represented as "senseless") are considered distinct forms of youth violence based on their location, victims, and alleged perpetrator (Bushman et al, 2016). While we acknowledge that the types of violence are distinct, we assert that the grieving caregiver, relative, or friend of an urban-residing youth killed by gun violence also wonders about the "sense" of the violent, young death even if they cognitively understand aspects of the circumstances associated with the death (Duck, 2009). Rather than speculate on the relative "sense" behind the violence, this phenomenological approach moves beyond reductionist representations of the causes and effects of violence. Beyond labels of "senselessness", it promotes multi–causal and varied sense–making around the interconnected and multiple layers of context of violence (Giorgi, 2004). In other words, a phenomenological approach seeks to explore the potential disparate as well as interconnected personal and contextual factors surrounding violence, thus contributing to sense-making without condoning or rationalizing a particular action. Using an applied and relational developmental systems scientific approach provides a contextual life-span perspective in order to address the pressing problems faced by individuals and society (R. M. Lerner, 2002; R. M. Lerner, Lerner, Bowers, & Geldhof, 2015), including senseless violence and victimization.

### *Psychological Perspective of a Victim or Survivor*

Although unpacking the meaning of an act of violence includes trying to ascertain the intent of the person carrying out the violent act, we begin with the target of the act. We begin with the survivor given that a considerable aspect of the trauma is in coping with the "senselessness" of the violence and is not limited to the practical matters associated with dealing with the violence itself. Although survivors are directly implicated by the event, a broader population of children and adults are negatively and indirectly affected given the lasting and deleterious effects on individuals who become aware of the violent acts, often as informed by the media (Jipguep & Sanders-Phillips, 2003). When people become aware of innocent victims, they ask themselves general questions like, "Why did this happen?" or, "What is the sense of this violence?" More personally, though, they may worry, "This could have been me" (Van Zomeren & Lodewijkx, 2009). This shift from concern for the general well-being of others to a specific worry for self–preservation marks an interesting transition in the intention of the bystander: while violence prevention may be portrayed as promoting social justice and eradicating oppression that may affect all people, gestures to alleviate violence may actually embody particular types of self-preservation.

While the motivation for self–preservation is folded into contemporary discourse that unpacks mass and "random" acts of violence, it is not a new argument. The 17th century English philosopher Thomas Hobbes (1894/1999) outlined what he considered natural laws that describe human behavior and postulated that individuals are motivated by the fear of their own violent death, and not the noble goals of seeking to promote peace, establish justice, or preserve lives or enhance their quality. Following this line of reasoning, then, violence that is legally prohibited (e.g., hate crimes associated with race, sexuality, or religion) may not always be described as "senseless" because some individuals may justify them given their own personal, political, social, or religious beliefs. As a result, while hate crimes may be considered abhorrent, there is rarely as widespread of a public outcry or broad political reaction as when violent acts are committed against a general cross-section of the population. When hearing of a hate crime directed at "someone else," individuals who are not members of the targeted groups may think, "That's too bad," but may not feel an urgent sense to preserve themselves (or by extension, their in-group) as they do not feel an imminent threat, and may also sense apathy towards out-group members, particularly members of lower-status groups (Arendt, 1970; Huddy, 2004).

An alternative perspective to a violent worldview assumes a more humanistic one grounded in a notion of a just world. A just world perspective assumes that individual actions are inherently inclined towards being morally fair and that noble actions are rewarded and evil ones are punished through a universal force that restores moral balance (M. J. Lerner, 1980, 1998). A just world perspective is compatible with a sense of interconnectedness or "cosmic connectedness" between diverse individuals, as opposed to perspectives where violence and self/in-group preservation are foundational. Within the just world literature, there are two sub-groups: one with belief in a just world towards self and the other with belief in a just world towards others. A study of 233 undergraduate psychology students found that belief in a just world to self was uniquely associated with numerous indicators for psychological health, while belief in a just world to others was uniquely related to harsh attitudes toward the poor which were not attributable to third influences or causes (Sutton & Douglas, 2005). While a just world perspective encompasses the agency of the individual, the universal moral force primarily engineers restorative justice, rather than individual and collective efforts to intentionally work to dismantle oppression and establish justice (Freire 1994/1970). A review of the literature on the just world perspective focuses on both the negative consequences as well as the psychological benefits of the belief, while addressing psychometrically improved measures that have identified cultural and demographic differences in the distribution of a just world perspective and its relation to victim blaming (Furnham, 2003). In addition, individual consciousness and orientation toward others varies according to multiple factors, including the content and form of our socialization messages.

## *Media and Social Messages Affecting the Sensibility of Violence*

An individual co-constructs their psychological outlook through the socialization influences that affect the individual, particularly the pervasive images in the media (Dubow, Huesmann, & Greenwood, 2007). A history of scholarship on the media outlines how the media creates racialized and often gendered portrayals of villains, frequently depicting them as male, non-White, and often Muslim (Saeed, 2008). These images may play an integral role in perception-making processes, including how our media viewing socializes us towards differentiated expectations based on social position. The media representations often depict people of color negatively (e.g., criminally, violently, and lazily). Consequently, these portrayals of people of color may lead to perceptions that people of color are as they are portrayed (i.e., negatively). Negative perceptions of a group play a role in the attribution of causality in acts of violence, particularly in determining the deservedness or sensibility behind the violence or the innocence of a victim. To illustrate, in Norway 35 first year psychology undergraduates and 49-non student individuals who varied in their college attendance and vocations participated in a controlled experiment to understand issues of blame-worthiness and victim attributes (Lodewijkx, Wildschut, Nijstad, Savenije, & Smit, 2001). The participants were given a brief newspaper report about an assault by one person, but with varied conditions regarding the details of the assault (e.g., the victim's prior engagement with the individual, both parties being involved in an argument). Participants were more likely to consider an act of violence as senseless and to identify with the victim when there was no opportunity to blame the victim, and when the victim had previously been uninvolved with the perpetrators.

How media presented and re-presented the event, then, affected viewers' "framing" of the event including the context of the assault and the assessment of blame, vulnerability, and purported randomness of the violence and relatedly the innocence or blameworthiness of the victim as well as the culpability or justification of the victimization agent (Van Zomeren & Lodewijkx, 2005). While the study of violence has roots in the sociocultural understanding of aggression and its situated meaning, the brevity of the sound-bite cycle generally leads to brief recapitulations of events that are decoupled from contextual details and their meaning from multiple stakeholders' varied perspectives. Such decontextualized depictions may not encompass the psychology and bio-ecological contexts of the victimizer and whether and how they may have been victimized earlier in their own life history, as well as their rationale in committing targeted or anonymous acts of violence (Bronfenbrenner & Morris, 2006). Therefore, in order to address the issue of violence holistically, we need to broaden the definition of senseless violence to include variations at the individual, social and structural levels and the relational dynamic between victim and victimizer.

### *Rethinking Sense Making Around Violence Through a Critical Developmental Approach*

In addition to broadening the understanding of violence to include sense-making surrounding the victims and their victimizers and the immediate and broader contexts that unite them, this manuscript seeks to problematize the dichotomy between violence that may seem "random" as well as others that seem to have a clearer, and relatedly, presumably preventable trajectory. For example, what is the sensibility surrounding interpersonal or relationship violence, particularly given the cyclical nature and the evidence that the abusers were often abused themselves? There is persistent evidence that experiencing abuse as a child has a range of negative effects on functioning long after the abuse stops, including chronic health problems, poor peer relations, delinquency and substance abuse during adolescence, and poor parenting as adults (Loeber and Farrington, 2012; Manly, Kim, Rogosch, & Cicchetti, 2001). Developmental pathways may be multiple and include neurobiological risk factors that are implicated due to either chronic or traumatic stress in adverse contexts during childhood that may alter the development of the brain (Bushman et al., 2016). In exploring the disproportional rates of homicidal and suicidal rates in males versus females, researchers across disciplines are beginning to unpack the narrow ways in which masculinity is defined in U.S. cultural contexts, rendering a crisis in human connection for males associated with unmet mental health needs (Representation Project, 2015; Way, 2013). For example, researchers documented all newspaper accounts of rampage school shootings in the United States between 1974–2002 and identified 25 incidents and 27 attackers; 85% of the attackers were White and male with average or better academic achievement, little history of school discipline, and with 78% characterized as socially marginalized (Newman et al., 2004). These varied examples of social disintegration surround a particular type of personal distress that is often invisible. The lack of public outcry or provision of material support to these silent victims beyond symbolic solidarity may explain the continuation of negative trajectories including violence towards self (e.g., substance use or abuse, engagement in risk behaviors, suicide) or violence toward others (e.g., abuse, assault, or homicide).

Rather than simply pointing fingers at individual culprits or victimizers, a broadened perspective on violence seeks to understand the complex socio-cultural factors that contribute to the violence, as well as to challenge our sensibilities around it. Imagine that instead of taking the lives of innocent people, the mass shooter shot a single bullet taking their own life. Would our sense of bewilderment be assuaged? Would we consider this just a "sad" story, but be glad there was no other "collateral damage," or would we even blame the individual for inflicting their own death? What if we learned that this shooter had been somehow victimized as a child, or had a history of mental illness, was marginalized or taunted regularly for some aspect of their identities, or was someone we knew and could have better supported as family or friends, neighbors, teachers, or psychologists? Our own culpability as well as the blame-worthiness of the victimizer can be further understood within more detailed sociological and psychological frameworks.

### *Developmental Contextualism as a Framework for Stratification and Violence*

The collective expression of violence is considered more rooted in the macro and micro social atmospheres of local to international social orders than in the individual personality traits of the victimizers (Blanco, Blanco, & Díaz, 2016). Understanding violence, then, requires understanding both the individual's development within their context (i.e., developmental contextualism, see Bronfenbrenner & Morris, 2006; R. M. Lerner, 2002; Rogoff, 2003; Super & Harkness, 1986). This theoretical model weaves anthropology, sociology, and psychology into a developmental model that includes the bi-directional influences between the individual and the multiple layers of context over time. Rather than considering contextual issues marginally, the current application anchors development within social stratification theory emphasizing the importance of racism, discrimination, oppression, and segregation on the developmental competencies of minoritized children and families as well as privileged ones (García Coll et al., 1996; Spencer, 2006). We will use developmental contextualism as a lens to understand the cyclical and multi-level nature of violence within the representation of minoritized individuals and groups within the law and higher education.

Given the highly stratified nature of social organizations and groups, scholars across disciplines have layered critical race and other critical theoretical perspectives to better understand the intersecting roles of race, gender, and other social positions on power. A critical race theoretical framework that applies a critical examination of society and culture to the intersection of race, law, and power, includes issues related to wealth and its distribution (Delgado & Stefancic, 2012). Within the United States and international contexts, issues of economic access and wealth accumulation are linked to historical realities such as slavery and colonialism that are manifest currently where an individual or group's level of advantage or disadvantage are highly correlated with their race (Fanon, 1963; Lareau & Conley, 2008). Just as wealth and property can be inherited, so can one's position as having relative (dis) advantage.

The critical analytic perspective to understanding the distribution of power across social groups has been extended to explore other dimensions of identity and how they intersect. In her seminal work, Crenshaw (1989) coined the term intersectionality and outlined how the legal system was limited to recognizing single axis issues of stratification (i.e., discrimination as either along race or gender groupings), thus overlooking the way race and gender may intersect and create complex layers where a single individual may occupy different layers of advantage or disadvantage based on the status of each social group of which they are members (i.e., White men, Black men, White women, and Black women). Within feminist scholarship and activism, the erasure of the identities of particular individuals by others who occupy positions of higher social, economic, and political power is considered an act of violence which many would consider senseless (Crenshaw, 1989), alongside the almost routine violence that shapes the lives of women and serves a particular social function (see Crenshaw, 1991 for references to related scholarship on the lives of battered women and the history of rape and coerced sexuality). This notion of intersectionality has been expanded and applied beyond legal contexts to a range of social justice issue to support advocacy along personal, social, and structural levels in a manner that recognizes individuals with complex and intersecting social positions along multiple axes (e.g., queer women of color, transgender women of color, non-binary people of color).

These systemic issues of stratification or violence lead to violence of different forms experienced at personal, social, and structural levels. For example, education and universities in particular are thought to be great equalizers contributing to social mobility in an egalitarian context that are particularly beneficial for those who are socially and economically most minoritized (Hout, 2012). While students with backgrounds from historically marginalized groups are increasingly gaining access to higher educational opportunities, their disproportional degree completion rates suggest that the focus on access needs to be expanded to include success, as measured by persistence and degree attainment (Brock, 2010), as well as the costs associated with the rising debt burden associated with college attendance. Lack of degree completion and other indicators related to tenure and promotion within higher education provide evidence of leaks in the academic pipeline along gendered fractures (Van Anders, 2004), as well as racial and class-based ones (Perna & Jones, 2013).

Within the broader conceptualization of access, success and persistence are often portrayed at the individual student level to describe proficiency in particular academic content and research skills. However, in coping with racism within higher educational contexts, persistence is described as a characteristic necessary for individuals to navigate structural and symbolic walls or barriers within institutional life (Ahmed, 2012), a type of collective violence against historically underrepresented and resilient student groups. In addition to the normative academic and psychological demands of higher education, then, students who are members of marginalized social groups (e.g., first generation, low income, and racial and ethnic minority college students, gender non-conforming, LGBTQA+) in higher education often face challenges of navigating unfamiliar, and often hostile, higher educational contexts (Lee & LaDousa, 2015). Consequently, a holistic focus on persistence should encompass both its academic dimensions, as well as its social and emotional aspects. To illustrate, when a female African American graduate student in chemistry sought support from her department chair to address her difficulties in forming a study group with her classmates partly because of how race affected peer dynamics, "…basically he told me, 'As department head there's nothing I can do…nothing I will do…nothing I should do. I really can't step in on these personal issues you are having.'" (Alexander & Herman, 2015, p. 9). While higher education institutions may have developed infrastructures to support diverse students (e.g., tutoring, financial aid packages that includes a laptop), this support may not capture the day-to-day challenges and acts of violence or omission that students face and affect their psychological functioning and well-being.

### Psychological Perspectives on Stratification and Violence

Within the large psychological umbrella, there are multiple theoretical and empirical ways to better understand the etiology and manifestations of violence. Continuing with the assumption that violence can be enacted at a micro-level, a psychological framing explores the social, developmental, and clinical ways in which we can understand violence.

### Internalizing Violent Vessages

How do our thoughts and feelings affect out behaviors, particularly towards in-group and out-group members? Often, we have been socialized in such tacit and cumulative ways, that we may be unconscious of and thus uncritical about our own socialization (Grusec & Hastings, 2014). These implicit messages get internalized in ways where we become less aware of power, thus unable to name problems associated with it, even when power is enacted inequitably (i.e., unjustly, oppressively, violently). A meta-analysis of fourteen million completed versions of the Implicit Association Test (IAT), where participants are asked to classify images of everyday objects or words, illustrates how the mind discriminates and provides evidence of bias towards White preference and equating being American with being White (Benaji & Greenwald, 2013). Gender versions of the same instrument confirmed multiple gender stereotypes (e.g., relative likelihood of a boss or surgeon associated with gender) (Benaji & Greenwald, 2013).

Even individuals who are members of nondominant social groups tend to prefer high status groups and negatively evaluate characteristics associated with their own social group (e.g., Blacks were likely to consider images related to Blacks unpleasant), suggesting an internalized oppression and the powerful effects of messages from the media and other socialization sources. Such negative evaluations are considered a type of mental health problem that is the result of racial stratification (Brown, 2003). Further, other research on skin color suggests higher levels of prejudice against individuals with darker skin tones and facial features and characteristics phenotypically associated with Blackness, so bias exists within and across racial groups (Maddox, 2004). Automatic cognitive evaluations based on implicit biases lead to inequitable treatment and behaviors at an interpersonal level (e.g., discomfort interacting with a Black student) as well as systemic ones (e.g., lost wages for women qualified to be surgeons or bosses), which are all types of violence.

Although implicit biases are thoughts, they may readily be translated into actions. On a concrete level, assumptions of guilt, blameworthiness, and criminality may affect individuals at critical moments of decisions, particularly while in a heightened state of arousal and armed with a weapon. Better understanding how the implicit biases of police officers responding to distress calls coupled with the social dominance orientation associated with their vocation, may help explain the rash of shootings by police of unarmed Black men in the United States and point to strategies to ameliorate the toxic situation (Hall, Hall, & Perry, 2016). Similarly, issues of bias and physical threat may affect how everyday citizens respond to one another in negotiating critical issues of safety and security in neighborhood contexts (Steele, 2010). To explore how racial and ethnic appearance may affect issues related to violence, a study with 78 Dutch participants examined which factors contributed to the labeling of violent incidents as "senseless" and found that if the act of violence was committed against a victim belonging to an ethnic minority (allochthonous victim), it was perceived to be more deserved and less senseless (and the desired penalty for the offender was smaller) than a similar violent act directed against a native (autochthonous) victim (Lodewijkx, Kwaadsteniet, & Nijstad, 2005). The preponderance of research that has found persistent implicit bias against Blacks has used images of adults, which is a problematic finding irrespective of age. Beyond Black men being viewed as menacing, White participants were asked to categorize threatening and nonthreatening objects (e.g., presentations of faces), and the collective findings across 4 experiments suggest that the perceived threat associated with Black men generalizes to young Black boys (Todd, Thiem, & Neel, 2016). Violence prevention needs to address how to re–message the socialization of such damaging biases.

### *Developing Proocial and Antisocial Thoughts and Behaviors*
Depriving people, particularly children, of the innocence they are generally presumed would typically be considered deplorable. When individuals override their ethical standards to justify thoughts and behaviors outside their typical moral realm, they convince themselves that the moral standards they normally adhere to do not apply in a particular context, thus redirecting their moral agency in order to enact behaviors they would otherwise consider inhumane (Bandura, Barbaranelli, Caprara, & Pastorelli, 1996). Further, in dehumanizing and oppressing others individuals, they may sanctify their harmful behavior as serving worthy causes, thus allowing them to hurt others and absolving themselves of blame by displacing responsibility and blameworthiness (Bandura, 2015), instead of centering and working through the causes for their own fragility (DiAngelo, 2011).

Individuals develop and are disciplined on how to attend to or ignore difference and inequality through a variety of institutions, including academic ones. Historically, the field of developmental psychology focused on a-historical and context-eliminating perspectives. Because of the leadership of numerous scholars and participants, the field currently affords more attention to context and acknowledges its stratified nature (i.e., not strictly meritocratic) and that navigating these barriers is central to the identity and developmental processes of minoritized individuals and communities (e.g., García Coll et. al., 1996; Kağitçibaşi, 2007; Spencer, 2006). Developmentally and contextually sensitive perspectives allow understanding how patterns may develop over the life course of individuals and groups or cohorts, as well as across generations.

Understanding developmental processes helps explain how issues of violence can be passed across generations. While family histories generally focus on genetic heritability, there are social processes that can explain how culture is transmitted, inherited, and transformed from one generation to the next (Rogoff, 2003), including the culture of violence. Social processes including play inform the cultural inheritance of introducing violence through everyday practices and objects, such as through violent toys and media (e.g., cartoons and video games). Nonverbal and language-based interactions with these objects, transmit socialization messages such that the content of violent messages may be internalized, normalized as being acceptable, and sometimes even deserved. Basic psychological studies show that even viewing the beating of a doll provides a model of violence that children later imitate when they were alone (Bandura, Ross, & Ross, 1963) and evidence has mounted with similar findings regarding increased aggression and desensitization through prolonged exposure to violence through television (Anderson & Bushman, 2002) as well as violent video games (Carnagey, Anderson, & Bushman, 2007). In addition, some children are explicitly taught that if someone hits or hurts you, to hit them back.

Violence for children is not only symbolically communicated, but can be experienced materially. Children not only learn about violence, but may be survivors of it through experiencing abuse or bullying by peers and siblings, as well as by a range of adults such as caregivers, teachers, and guardians. The violence may take multiple forms, and include emotional, verbal, sexual, and physical forms of abuse. It may be further complicated by other stressors, including poverty, living in a context with high levels of neighborhood violence, and addiction. Healing the survivor's emotional needs is a complex process and may not be guaranteed. Through modeling of violence, especially when coupled with no or ineffective intervention to stop the violence, the bullied may become the bullier, and thus continue the cycle of violence at an interpersonal level. In many cases the primary focus is on how to promote individual resilience and coping, which is important. In addition, though, there needs to be a parallel and systemic focus on how to reduce toxic messages and behaviors (i.e., help the bullier stop bullying, not just making the bullied a more resilient target).

### *Indications of Maladaptive Development or Trajectories*
Both traumatic experiences as well as chronic experiences of stressors of varied forms may contribute to clinical psychological issues. The injustices may be acute and enduring artifacts of systemic violence, such as the relationship between colonialism and mental illness (Fanon, 1963; Hickling & Hutchinson, 2000). They may also include the barrage of constant minor stressors, as in the case of microaggressions. Microaggressions are subtle forms of bias and discrimination that are perpetuated by dominant or privileged groups or individuals, often unintentionally and related to one's implicit biases (Sue et al., 2007). Microaggressions may alienate individuals who represent a range of social groups (e.g., race, gender, sexuality), but share being marginalized in some way because of their social position. Although comments may seem innocuous (e.g., he doesn't belong, they don't have anything in common), they contain denigrating messages; managing these messages saps the psychological and spiritual energy of recipients (Sue et al., 2007; Sue, 2010). The cumulative effects of microaggressions and other types of life stress (e.g., discrimination, chronic poverty) have been found to contribute to premature aging and health risks (e.g., depression, compromised immunity) as evidenced by the accelerated shortening of telomere length for individuals experiencing chronic stress (Chae et al., 2014; Epel et al., 2004).

Considering psychological well-being, at least some portion of how victims and victimizers develop is not what they have become, but what their current level of status and power ascribes or enables them to be. Part of the ambiguity of these processes and outcomes may reflect the fluidity of situations and managing conflicting expectations across contexts. Although often studied within the context of war veterans struggling to come to terms with the violence they may have witnessed or been compelled to execute, morally injurious events include perpetrating, failing to prevent, or witnessing acts that transgress deeply held moral beliefs (Litz et al., 2009). This betrayal of "what's right" by a person in authority or by oneself is deemed a potentially injurious moral event and has been found to impair the capacity for trust, elevate despair, and increase levels of both personal and interpersonal violence (Shay, 2014). Although the situation may not be one of combat, individuals who are members of maligned social groups and mistreated personally and marginalized both socially and structurally are in a different type of battle and may suffer moral injury because of unjust treatment. These injustices may deleteriously affect their coping and psychological well-being (e.g., through self-injurious behaviors, poor mental health, suicide ideation), as well as relations with others (e.g., externalizing behaviors, homicidal ideation).

### Human Geography and the Migration of Violence

While critical race theory has contributed to providing a framework for multi–axis social identities, it has been critiqued for romanticizing a focus grounded in present and future social configurations, with a complacent amnesia regarding how complex histories continue to form racial and other social configurations and geographies (Mahtani, 2014). The literature on human geography focuses on how violence against individuals is inflicted on bodies; individuals who transport and embody violence in their interactions, thus connecting violence through people across time and space. The study of human geography explores the interaction between human beings and their environment and includes a range of issues including the ways in which health and economic resources are informed by geographic factors and distributed unevenly (Gregory, Johnston, Pratt, Watts, & Whatmore, 2011). The way in which individuals and groups interact with the environment provides a person-centered framing for understanding stratification and the violence embedded within it. For example, because sexual violence disproportionately affects women, the study of human geography integrates geography and feminist analyses (Hyndman, 2004; Pain, 1991). Micro, meso, and macro structural violences are experienced by individuals at the scale of the body. Furthermore, bodies move through spaces that create and inform climate and space. To illustrate, a participatory action research (PAR) study of micro-aggressions at an elite college campus challenged the notions of knowledge production by providing an opportunity to document and reflect on one's personal experiences and locate how they are embedded in social and structural contexts through an interactive art installation where individuals could reflect on microaggressions that they produce and receive (Abo-Zena & Pavalow, 2016). The multiple perspectives surrounding social disorder and psychosocial trauma that were reflected in the PAR study are captured in a framework that posits that the widespread prevalence of interpersonal and collective violence would benefit from looking earlier, outside, and beyond the person's mental health in order to understand the mutually constitutive interactions between the individual and the macro and micro contextual actors and forces (Blanco et al., 2016). Better understanding how violence in its many forms moves across individuals and geographical landscapes is important in order to understand how individuals are related to their contexts and their other relationships, which may help reconcile enduring rifts within relationships and dismantle violence.

### Discussion, Implications, and Conclusion

Given that the relational connection between victim and victimizer contributes to the "sense" and "senselessness" of violent acts, it is important to explore the multiple ways in which they are connected. Freire (1994/1970) describes the mirror relationship between the oppressed and the oppressor and the iterative manner in which, when given the opportunity, the oppressed often assumes the practices and values of the oppressor unless involved in a critical reflection on values and actions. In large part, this behavior may reflect a dimension of the Hobbesian notion of self-preservation (i.e., given a social structure built on inequality, a previously oppressed person would seek to protect their self-interest and oppress others instead of be oppressed).

Ironically, though, this attempt to preserve oneself is an act of self–sabotage: Freire (1994/ 1970) describes the process of oppressing others as a dehumanizing one because it objectifies the oppressed person and renders the oppressor as lacking humanity. Furthermore, the precarious social situation characterized by its inequity and oppression jeopardizes the well-being of the oppressed and the oppressor, as evidenced throughout history by examples of loss of life, liberty, and property in the quest for individuals, tribes, groups, or nations to assert their humanity. Finally, in addition to the oppressor's constantly needing to be on the defensive because of their offenses, the act of oppressing others makes the oppressor at risk for feeling guilty. For the victim and the victimizer, there are numerous and interrelated costs that are both internalized (e.g., guilt, resentment) as well as externalized (e.g., micro- and macro aggressions, assaults, and other forms of violence).

In order to move from a framework where we pay heavy individual and societal tolls around the violence we fear, witness, or experience, we need to develop an alternative framework to establish peace and eliminate oppression. We need to adopt a pedagogy for the oppressed (which includes us all, in some way at some time) from the oppressor (which includes us all, in some way at some time) (Freire, 1994/1970). This includes diverse stakeholders who operate from different disciplines and types of work to collaborate together (e.g., activists, organizers, researchers, practitioners, entrepreneurs, workers) to highlight strategies and approaches to better recognize inequalities in their many forms (e.g., disproportionately or lack of representation of women and people of color in business or STEM, water and refugee "crises"). As problematic issues are documented, we need to develop systems and strategies to address them, such as efforts to expand the "canon" of fundamental scholarship to be more inclusive of the experiences and histories of diverse scholars and people and peoples. Starting with higher educational institutions, we can explore the person-centered and other molecular ways in which violence may be reflected throughout the curriculum and academic offerings, extracurricular offerings, and student life and general campus climate in order to document how policies and practices may be informed by and respond to people's personal and collective experiences and needs on college campuses (e.g., soaring costs, unmet mental health needs, limited employment prospects post-graduation). In particular, coursework and other scholarship should explicitly consider the interconnected nature of violence and relationship between victim and victimizer. In applied contexts, social justice work should be linked to critical theory and critical human geographies in a reciprocal relationship where theory is regularly linked to some form of engaged practice, thus explicitly connecting reflections on past to forming present and future possibilities. Beyond higher education, we should promote similar multifaceted and integrated inquiry-action campaigns within workplaces, neighborhoods, community organizations, military, and the media.

This paper has sought to re-define the term "senseless violence" to include both large scale attacks that seem to be directed at "random" targets, thus lacking "sense" in their method, but also to question the apparent and hidden sources of aggressors and aggression to include externalized and internalized manifestations of violence, against targeted and random groups as well as targeted and random individuals. The targets may reflect in-group and out-group members and also may include the self. Wherever we look, we see prolific evidence of violence at almost every sub-culture of society (e.g., bullying in schools has expanded to the even more prolific cyber bullying and public shaming, substance abuse and addictions, mental illness, self-injury, homicide), but we also see random and organized acts of kindness and advocating for justice.

The interconnected nature (but disconnected representation) of the aggression, aggressors, and sources of stressors are part of the system that perpetuate the violence, and make its experience feel isolating to the direct and indirect victims. Consider a college student who died of an overdose. The parents were in communication with their son and know of his addiction, but unaware of the severity of the problem. The University was aware of the addiction, but underestimated the problem. The parents arrived for a campus visit to find their son dead and alone. All lament that his death was preventable and that his coping and suffering were isolated. Connecting the dots between the personal, social, and structural sources and manifestations of violence may better illustrate the connectedness between victim and victimizers, causes and effects of violence, and thus better allow us to disrupt the cycles of violence and re–place the connections in a manner that reduces violence through humanizing ourselves and others.

## References

Abo-Zena, M. M., & Pavalow, M. (2016). Being In-Between Participatory Action Research as a Tool to Partner With and Learn About Emerging Adults. *Emerging Adulthood, 4*(1), 19–29.

Ahmed, S. (2012). *On being included: Racism and diversity in institutional life.* Durham, NC: Duke University Press.

Aitken, S. C. (2001). Schoolyard shootings: Racism, sexism, and moral panics over teen violence. *Antipode, 33*(4), 593–600.

Alexander, Q. R., & Hermann, M. A. (2015). African-American women's experiences in graduate science, technology, engineer, and mathematics education at a predominantly white university: A qualitative investigation. *Journal of Diversity in Higher Education*, Online first publication. http://dx.doi.org/10.1037//a0039705.

Anderson, C. A., & Bushman, B. J. (2002). The effects of media violence on society. *Science, 295*(5564), 2377–2379.

Arendt, H. (1970). *On violence.* Boston, MA: Houghton Mifflin Harcourt.

Banaji, M. R., & Greenwald, A. G. (2013). *Blindspot: Hidden biases of good people.* New York, NY: Delacorte Press.

Bandura, A. (2015). *Moral disengagement: How people do harm and live with themselves.* New York, NY: Worth.

Bandura, A., Ross, D., & Ross, S. A. (1963). Imitation of film-mediated aggressive models. *The Journal of Abnormal and Social Psychology, 66*(1), 3–11.

Bandura, A., Barbaranelli, C., Caprara, G. V., & Pastorelli, C. (1996). Mechanisms of moral disengagement in the exercise of moral agency. *Journal of Personality and Social Psychology, 71*(2), 364.

Blanco, A., Blanco, R., & Díaz, D. (2016). Social (dis) order and psychosocial trauma: Look earlier, look outside, and look beyond the persons. *American Psychologist, 71*(3), 187–198.

Blok, A. (2000). The enigma of senseless violence. In G. Aijmer & J. Abbink (Eds.), *Meanings of violence: A cross cultural perspective* (pp. 23–38). New York, NY: New York University Press.

Brock, T. (2010). Young adults and higher education: Barriers and breakthroughs to success. *Transition to adulthood, 20*(1), 109–132. Retrieved from https://www.princeton.edu/futureofchildren/publications/journals/article/index.xml?journ.

Bronfenbrenner, U., & Morris, P. A. (2006). The bioecological model of human development. *Handbook of child psychology*. In W. Overton, P. Molenaar, & R. M. Lerner (Eds.), *Handbook of child psychology and developmental science: Vol. 1. Theory and method* (7th ed., pp. 793–828). Hoboken, NJ: Wiley.

Brown, T. N. (2003). Critical race theory speaks to the sociology of mental health: Mental health problems produced by racial stratification. *Journal of Health and Social Behavior, 44*(3), 292–301.

Bushman, B. J., Newman, K., Calvert, S. L., Downey, G., Dredze, M., Gottfredson, M., & Romer, D. (2016). Youth violence: What we know and what we need to know. *American Psychologist, 71*(1), 17–39.

Carnagey, N. L., Anderson, C. A., & Bushman, B. J. (2007). The effect of video game violence on physiological desensitization to real-life violence. *Journal of Experimental Social Psychology, 43*(3), 489–496.

Chae, D. H., Nuru-Jeter, A. M., Adler, N. E., Brody, G. H., Lin, J., Blackburn, E. H., & Epel, E. S. (2014). Discrimination, racial bias, and telomere length in African-American men, *American Journal of Preventive Medicine, 46*(2), 103–11, http://dx.doi.org/10.1016/j.amepre.2013.10.020

Chiricos, T., & Eschholz, S. (2002). The racial and ethnic typification of crime and the criminal typification of race and ethnicity in local television news. *Journal of Research in Crime and Delinquency, 39*(4), 400–420.

Coll, C. G., Lamberty, G., Jenkins, R., McAdoo, H. P., Crnic, K., Wasik, B. H., & Garcia, H. V. (1996). An integrative model for the study of developmental competencies in minority children. *Child Development, 67*(5), 1891–1914.

Crary, J. (2013). *24/7: Late capitalism and the ends of sleep*. New York, NY: Verso Books.

Crenshaw, K. (1989). Demarginalizing the intersection of race and sex: A black feminist critique of antidiscrimination doctrine, feminist theory and antiracist politics. *University of Chicago Legal Forum, 1989*(1),139–168.

Crenshaw, K. (1991). Mapping the margins: Intersectionality, identity politics, and violence against women of color. *Stanford Law Review*, 1241–1299.

Delgado, R., & Stefancic, J. (2012). *Critical race theory: An introduction*. New York, NY: NYU Press.

DiAngelo, R. (2011). White fragility. *The International Journal of Critical Pedagogy, 3*(3), 54–70.

Dubow, E. F., Huesmann, L. R., & Greenwood, D. (2007). Media and youth socialization: Underlying process and moderators of effects (pp. 404–430). In J. E. Grusec & P. D. Hastings (Eds.), *Handbook of socialization: Theory and research*. New York, NY: Guilford Press.

Duck, W. (2009). 'Senseless' violence: Making sense of murder. *Ethnography, 10*(4), 417–434.

Epel, E. S., Blackburn, E. H., Lin, J., Dhabhar, F. S., Adler, N. E., Morrow, J. D., & Cawthon, R. M. (2004). Accelerated telomere shortening in response to life stress. *Proceedings of the National Academy of Sciences of the United States of America, 101*(49), 17312–17315

Fanon, F. (1963). *The wretched of the earth*. Translated by Constance Farrington. New York, NY: Grove Press.

Freire, P. (1994/1970). *Pedagogy of the oppressed*. New York, NY: Continuum Publishing.

Furnham, A. (2003). Belief in a just world: Research progress over the past decade. *Personality and individual differences, 34*(5), 795–817.

Giorgi, A. (2004). A way to overcome the methodological vicissitudes involved in researching subjectivity. *Journal of Phenomenological Psychology, 35*(1), 1–25.

Gregory, D., Johnston, R., Pratt, G., Watts, M., & Whatmore, S. (Eds.). (2011). *The dictionary of human geography*. Singapore: Wiley.

Grusec, J. E., & Hastings, P. D. (Eds.). (2014). *Handbook of socialization: Theory and research*. New York: Guilford.

Hall, A. V., Hall, E. V., & Perry, J. L. (2016). Black and blue: Exploring racial bias and law enforcement in the killings of unarmed black male civilians. *American Psychologist, 71*(3), 175–186.

Hickling, F. W., & Hutchinson, G. (2000). Post-colonialism and mental health. *Psychiatric Bulletin*, *24*, 94–95.

Hobbes, T. (1894/1999). *Leviathan: Or, the matter, form, and power of a commonwealth ecclesiastical and civil* (Vol. 21). New York: G. Routledge and Sons.

Hout, M. (2012). Social and economic returns to college education in the United States. *Annual Review of Sociology*, *38*, 379–400.

Huddy, L. (2004). Contrasting theoretical approaches to intergroup relations. *Political Psychology*, *25* (6), 947–967. Retrieved from http://www.jstor.org/stable/3792284

Hyndman, J. (2004). Mind the gap: bridging feminist and political geography through geopolitics. *Political Geography*, *23*(3), 307–322.

Jipguep, M., & Sanders-Phillips, K. (2003). The context of violence for children of color: Violence in the community and in the media. *The Journal of Negro Education*, *72*(4), 379–395. Retrieved from http://www.jstor.org/stable/3211190

Kağitçibaşi, C. (2007). *Family, self, and human development* (2nd ed.). Mahwah, NJ: Erlbaum.

King, M. L. Jr. (1958/2010). *Stride toward freedom: the Montgomery Story*. Boston, MA: Beacon Press.

Lareau, A., & Conley, D. (Eds.) (2008). *Social class: How does it work?*. New York, NY: Russell Sage.

Lee, E. M. & LaDousa, C. (2015). *College students' experiences of power and marginality: Sharing spaces and negotiating differences*. New York, NY: Routledge.

Lerner, M. J. (1980). *The belief in a just world*. New York, NY: Springer US.

Lerner, M. J. (1998). *The two forms of belief in a just world*. New York, NY: Springer US.

Lerner, R. M. (2002). *Concepts and theories of human development* (3rd ed.). Mahwah, NJ: Erlbaum.

Lerner, R. M., Lerner, J. V., Bowers, E., & Geldhof, G. J. (2015). Positive youth development: A relational developmental systems model. In W. Overton, P. Molenaar, & R. M. Lerner (Eds.), *Handbook of child psychology and developmental science: Vol. 1. Theory and method* (7th ed., pp. 607–651). Hoboken, NJ: Wiley.

Li, S. C. (2003). Biocultural orchestration of developmental plasticity across levels: the interplay of biology and culture in shaping the mind and behavior across the life span. *Psychological Bulletin*, *129*(2), 171–194.

Litz, B. T., Stein, N., Delaney, E., Lebowitz, L., Nash, W. P., Silva, C., & Maguen, S. (2009). Moral injury and moral repair in war veterans: A preliminary model and intervention strategy. *Clinical psychology review*, *29*(8), 695–706.

Lodewijkx, H. F., Kwaadsteniet, E. W., & Nijstad, B. A. (2005). That could be me (or not): Senseless violence and the role of deservingness, victim ethnicity, person identification, and position identification. *Journal of Applied Social Psychology*, *35*(7), 1361–1383.

Lodewijkx, H. F. M., Wildschut, T., Nijstad, B. A., Savenije, W., & Smit, M. (2001). In a violent world a just world makes sense: The case of "senseless violence" in the Netherlands. *Social Justice Research*, *14*(1), 79–94.

Loeber, R., & Farrington, D. P. (2012). *From juvenile delinquency to adult crime: Criminal careers, justice policy and prevention*. New York, NY: Oxford University Press.

Maddox, K. B. (2004). Perspectives on racial phenotypicality bias. *Personality and Social Psychology Review*, *8*(4), 383-401.

Mahtani, M. (2014). Toxic geographies: Absences in critical race thought and practice in social and cultural geography. *Social & Cultural Geography*, *15*(4), 359–367.

Manly, J. T., Kim, J. E., Rogosch, F. A., & Cicchetti, D. (2001). Dimensions of child maltreatment and children's adjustment: Contributions of developmental timing and subtype. *Development and Psychopathology*, *13*(04), 759–782.

Newman, K. S., Fox, C., Harding, D., & Mehta, J. (2004). *Rampage: The social roots of school shootings*. New York, NY: Basic Books.

Newsom, J. S., Congdon, J., & Anthony, J. (Producers) & Newsom, J. (Director) (2015), *The mask you live in* [Documentary]. IMDpro.

Pain, R. (1991). Space, sexual violence and social control: Integrating geographical and feminist analyses of women's fear of crime. *Progress in Human Geography*, *15*(4), 415–431.

Perna, L., & Jones A. (2013). *The state of college access and completion: Improving college success for students from underrepresented groups*. New York, NY: Routledge.

Representation Project (2015). The mask you live in. Retrieved from http://therepresentationproject.org/

Rogoff, B. (2003). *The cultural nature of human development*. New York, NY: Oxford University Press.

Saeed, A. (2008). Teaching and earning guide for media, racism and Islamophobia: The representation of Islam and Muslims in the media. *Sociology Compass, 2*(6), 2041–2047.

Schmidt, B., & Schröder, I. (2001). *Anthropology of violence and conflict*. New York, NY: Routledge.

Shay, J. (2014). Moral injury. *Psychoanalytic Psychology, 31*(2), 182–191. doi:org/10.1037/a0036090

Spencer, M. B. (2006). Phenomenology and ecological systems theory: Development of diverse groups. In W. Damon & R. M. Lerner (Eds.). *Handbook of child psychology: An advanced textbook* (pp. 829–893). Hoboken, NJ: Wiley.

Staudigl, M. (2007). Towards a phenomenological theory of violence: Reflections following Merleau-Ponty and Schutz. *Human Studies, 30*(3), 233–253. Retrieved from http://www.jstor.org/stable/27642795

Steele, C. M. (2010). *Whistling Vivaldi*. New York, NY: Norton.

Sue, D. W. (2010). *Microaggressions in everyday life: Race, gender, and sexual orientation*. Hoboken, NJ: Wiley.

Sue, D. W., Capodilupo, C. M., Torino, G. C., Bucceri, J. M., Holder, A., Nadal, K. L., & Esquilin, M. (2007). Racial microaggressions in everyday life: Implications for clinical practice. American Psychologist, 62 (4), 271–286. doi:org/10.1037/0003-066X.62.4.271

Super, C. M., & Harkness, S. (1986). The developmental niche: A conceptualization at the interface of child and culture. *International Journal of Behavioral Development, 9*(4), 545–569.

Sutton, R. M., & Douglas, K. M. (2005). Justice for all, or just for me? More evidence of the importance of the self-other distinction in just-world beliefs. *Personality and Individual Differences, 39*(3), 637–645.

Todd, A. R., Thiem, K. C., & Neel, R. (2016). Does seeing faces of young black boys facilitate the identification of threatening stimuli? *Psychological Science, 27*(3), 384–393.

Van Anders, S. M. (2004). Why the academic pipeline leaks: Fewer men than women perceive barriers to becoming professors. *Sex Roles, 51*(9-10), 511–521.

Van Zomeren, M., & Lodewijkx, H. F. (2005). Motivated responses to 'senseless' violence: Explaining emotional and behavioral responses through person and position identification. *European Journal of Social Psychology, 35*(6), 755–766.

Van Zomeren, M., & Lodewijkx, H. F. (2009). "Could this happen to me?": Threat related state orientation increases position identification with victims of random, "senseless" violence. *European Journal of Social Psychology, 39*(2), 223–236.

Vasterman, P. L. (2005). Media-hype self-reinforcing news waves, journalistic standards and the construction of social problems. *European Journal of Communication, 20*(4), 508–530.

Way, N. (2013). *Deep secrets: Boys' friendships and the crisis of connection*. Cambridge, MA: Harvard University Press.

# In Search of Meaning: Are School Rampage Shootings Random and Senseless Violence?

Eric Madfis

**ABSTRACT**

This article discusses Joel Best's (1999) notion of random violence and applies his concepts of pointlessness, patternlessness, and deterioration to the reality about multiple-victim school shootings gleaned from empirical research about the phenomenon. Best describes how violence is rarely random, as scholarship reveals myriad observable patterns, lots of discernable motives and causes, and often far too much fear-mongering over how bad society is getting and how violent we are becoming. In contrast, it is vital that the media, scholars, and the public better understand crime patterns, criminal motivations, and the causes of fluctuating crime rates. As an effort toward such progress, this article reviews the academic literature on school rampage shootings and explores the extent to which these attacks are and are not random acts of violence.

"School shootings are always incomprehensible and horrific tragedies…" -Education Secretary Arne Duncan after the 2012 shooting at Sandy Hook Elementary School in Connecticut (Wolfgang, 2012)

"The prevalence of gun violence in this country is a sickness that continues to claim innocent lives and threaten our communities seemingly at random on a daily basis…We have seen too many of these pointless, brutal tragedies." -New York Governor Andrew Cuomo after the 2015 shooting at Umpqua Community College in Oregon (Velasquez, 2015)

It is not uncommon to perceive school rampage shootings, often defined as incidents in which one or more shooters attack their current or former school and kill multiple victims (Newman, Fox, Roth, Mehta, & Harding, 2004), as random, nonsensical, and/or senseless acts of violence. Some scholars (Kimmel & Mahler, 2003; Volokh, 2000) characterize school rampage shootings as "random" events at least in part because of the much touted (though empirically questionable) notion that school rampage shooters attack peers and teachers in an indiscriminate manner without deliberate targets in mind. In fact, the presence of random victims is often used as an operational criterion in defining rampage shootings. For example, Newman and her colleagues (2004) specifically limit their definition of school rampage to include only those cases in which at least some of the victims were chosen randomly or symbolically. Likewise, Muschert (2007) distinguishes "targeted" school shootings with multiple specifically intended victims from "rampage" school shootings which necessitate random or symbolic victims. More generally, rampage attacks in schools have been described as "non-sensical" (Wike & Fraser, 2009, p. 167) and "senseless" (Solomon, 2014; Molinet, 2014) due to an assumption that they are motiveless or unexplainable. Additionally, it is far too frequently assumed that these deadly incidents are a completely new phenomenon of contemporary society or one which is now occurring with unprecedented frequency.

In fact, all of these problematic assumptions fit directly in line with what Joel Best (1999) critiques as the problematic construct of patternless and pointless "random violence." Perfect statistical randomness occurs when no discernible patterns exist at all. While media often depict violence and other crimes this way, violence is not really so random, confusing, and unknowable. In his book *Random Violence: How We Talk about New Crimes and New Victims*, Best focuses on three different aspects of how the media mistakenly portrays violence to be random: violence as patternless, violence as pointless, and violence as deterioration.

Violence may be considered patternless when it could happen to anyone at any time and when everyone is equally likely to be both a perpetrator and victim of violence. However, it is inaccurate when the media depict violence as lacking any noticeable patterns. In fact, research on violence indicates that there are many typical and discernable social patterns (i.e., violence is characteristically intra-racial, intra-class, and perpetrated by males) (Fox, Levin, & Quinet, 2012). While some crimes certainly result in random victims (such as when stray bullets strike unintended targets), by and large, it is not the case that everyone is equally likely to be an offender or a victim. Negative social experiences such as negative peer and family influences, poverty, substance abuse, mental illness, and many other issues certainly increase one's likelihood of becoming a violent offender and/or a victim of a violent crime (Best, 1999; Lanier, Stuart, & Desire, 2015; Fox et al., 2012).

The second aspect of depicting violence as random is the issue of pointlessness. Violence is conceived as pointless when it is assumed to occur for no reason at all, without any intended purpose or rational motive on the part of violent offenders. Best (1999) argues that it is problematic and incorrect for media to depict violent acts as lacking any discernible point or meaning. Of course, the senseless loss of human life is always "pointless," but there is usually a purpose or goal behind violent actions, at least from the offender's perspective. People do not typically just commit crimes for no reason, even if their reasoning is difficult for law abiding people to understand (Best, 1999; Fox et al., 2012). To simply state that a particular violent act is "just the kind of things that *those* types of people do" is not helpful; it does not explain the true causes of violence, and it does not help prevent future incidents. To understand violence, we must view people's actions from their own point-of-view in line with Max Weber's (1978) notion of "verstehen," which refers to the process in which an outside observer of a culture attempts to subjectively and empathetically relate to it and understand it in terms of situated meaning and experience. Accordingly, it is important to investigate how seemingly irrational and pointless crimes may be rational and meaningful for offenders (as in Ferrell's 1997 concept of "criminological verstehen"). To understand behavior from the perspective of offenders is to see that they do typically have a purpose for their actions; it is not merely pointless to them.

The third aspect of depicting violence as random is the issue of deterioration. This refers to the mistaken idea that society is continually getting worse and rates of violent crime are always increasing over time. In fact, in recent years, the United States has seen a remarkable decrease in both crime, in general, and violent crime, in particular. The highest crime rate in U.S. history occurred during the early 1990s, but it has steadily declined since that time

(Conklin, 2002; Fox & Burstein, 2010). It is certainly possible we are currently experiencing a temporary reprieve and the crime rate will increase again, but the salient point is that there is always fluctuation; society is certainly not inevitably and continuously deteriorating with increased violence. In fact, when summarizing his expansive historical analysis of violence over millennia, Harvard psychologist Steven Pinker (2007) argues that violence has declined remarkably over the course of human history and that "today we are probably living in the most peaceful moment of our species' time on earth."

Best's (1999) three problematic tropes are often applied to the phenomenon of rampage school shootings. The pervasive misperception that school rampages are random acts of violence encourages people to think that there are no recognizable patterns in terms of whom the victims and offenders of this crime are and that there are no commonalities regarding the types of schools and communities which have disproportionately been attacked. Perceived randomness also serves to obfuscate genuine identifiable causes and offender motivations. Further, the random label distorts and exaggerates the level of risk in society and increases fear such that people believe rampage attacks are far more likely to occur than they actually are (Madfis, 2016). As such, this article will directly engage with Best's three critiques of randomness by utilizing empirical research to showcase the extent to which school rampage shootings are and are not random acts of violence.

## School Rampage as a Social Problem

Many recent tragedies (such as those at Sandy Hook Elementary School in Newtown, Connecticut, at the University of California, Santa Barbara, at Marysville Pilchuck High School in Washington State, and at Oregon's Umpqua Community College) have led media and the public to be increasingly aware of this particularly heinous crime. These events were highly publicized as they shocked the American public not only for their brutality, but because of the prior belief that such schools were "safe havens, free of the dangers of street crime" (Lawrence, 2007, p. 147). That such violence could be perpetrated in middle and upper class school districts away from the plight of impoverished urban areas has been perceived as especially perplexing (Kimmel & Mahler, 2003). Perhaps unsurprisingly, a great deal of empirical research has been conducted on the phenomenon in the last two decades (see Muschert, 2007; Rocque, 2012; Sommer, Leuschner, & Scheithauer, 2014 for fairly comprehensive reviews).

While the term "school shooting" has been defined and operationalized in numerous ways by many different scholars, Newman et al. (2004) can be credited with delineating the concept of "rampage school shootings," which "take place on a school-related public stage before an audience; involve multiple victims, some of whom are shot simply for their symbolic significance or at random; and involve one or more shooters who are students or former students of the school" (p. 50). While only a portion of school gun violence fits all of these criteria (and the overall majority of school homicides are single-victim), the most highly publicized events during the last two decades tend to conform to these specifics. In addition to the aforementioned rampage shootings, Muschert (2007, p. 62) has filled in this typological picture to form the accompanying school shooting categories of "mass murders" committed by older non-student perpetrators, "terrorist attacks" engaged in by individuals or groups to advance their political or ideological goals, "targeted shootings" that involve only specific pre-planned victims, and the "government shootings" of student protesters. For the purpose of this article, discussion will be limited to rampage school shootings with multiple victims committed by former or current students.

Many scholars (Aitken, 2001; Best, 2002; Burns & Crawford, 1999; Killingbeck, 2001; Madfis, 2016; Muschert & Peguero, 2010), have asserted that the recent American response to rampage school shootings has constituted a moral panic, in that the reaction has been based on an exaggerated perception of their pervasiveness, prevalence, and threat to social order bred by excesses in media coverage (Cohen, 2011). True as this may be, these events did genuinely occur with greater frequency in middle and high schools in the late 1990s (Fox et al., 2012) and then on college campuses in the late 2000s (Fox & Savage, 2009), and dozens of plots to commit such heinous crimes are revealed and pre-empted every year (Madfis, 2014a). Likewise, since the April 1999 Columbine massacre, school shooters across the country and in nations around the world have turned to this infamous American case for homicidal inspiration (Larkin, 2009; Madfis & Levin, 2013). Although school rampage attacks are extremely rare, these incidents warrant serious concern, for when they do occur, they not only cause multiple casualties, but leave many survivors and bystanders with post-traumatic stress (James, 2009; Schwarz & Kowalski, 1991) and create extensive fear among the larger public (Altheide, 2009; Burns & Crawford, 1999).

## School Rampages are not Pointless for Offenders

From the perspective of school rampage offenders, their crimes are anything but pointless and without motive. In search of the etiology of school rampage shootings, motivations have been explored by a vast array of academics ranging from sociologists and criminologists to anthropologists, social workers, psychologists, and psychiatrists. Often, scholars have brought one particular causal factor to the fore, whether it is the mental deficiency of individual perpetrators, the school or community context, or the larger socio-cultural background.

At the individual-level, some have focused on the mental illnesses and personality disorders of said killers (Langman, 2009a, 2009b; McGee & DeBernardo, 1999). While severe mental illnesses, such as schizophrenia and bipolar disorder are rare in mass killers in and out of school settings, a history of suicidal thoughts and depression are far more common (Fox & DeLateur, 2014; McGee & DeBernardo, 1999; Vossekuil, Fein, Reddy, Borum, & Modzeleski, 2002). That said, these mental health concerns themselves cannot fully explain these events, as most people with mental illnesses are not violent (Schug & Fradella, 2014), thus one must still strive to understand why someone with a mental health issue would desire to commit a rampage attack and not neglect external motivations.

At the micro-social interpersonal level, many have stressed the role played by negative relationships with peers, such as victimization through bullying (Burgess, Garbarino, & Carlson, 2006; Kimmel & Mahler, 2003; Klein, 2012; Larkin, 2007; Leary, Mark Kowalski, Smith, & Phillips, 2003; Levin & Madfis, 2009). Both the exclusionary nature of teenage cliques (Larkin, 2007; Lickel et al., 2003) and the cohesion of intolerant, homogeneous, and tightly knit communities (Aronson, 2004; Newman et al., 2004) have been implicated in previous rampage attacks.

At the macro-sociological level, various researchers have clarified the role that aggrieved masculinity (Kimmel & Mahler, 2003; Madfis, 2014c; Mai & Alpert, 2000), a desire for lasting fame (Lankford, 2016), and the widespread accessibility and acceptance of gun culture

(Glassner, 2010; Haider-Markel & Joslyn, 2001; Lawrence & Birkland, 2004; Webber, 2003) play in reinforcing and legitimizing violent solutions. As boys and men who have felt profoundly disempowered and emasculated, offenders often perceive that their commission of an infamous and widely-reported school attack with significant firepower and large body counts will regain their lost sense of masculinity, superiority, and power.

Of late, scholars (such as Henry, 2009; Hong, Cho, Allen-Meares, & Espelage, 2011; Levin & Madfis, 2009) have attempted to fuse these disparate etiological concerns to achieve a more multi-faceted, holistic, and cross-disciplinary understanding of the causes of school rampage across the micro, meso, and macro levels of analysis. Levin and Madfis' (2009) cumulative strain theory proposed a five-stage integrated and sequential model in which several criminological theories (strain theory, control theory, and routine activities theory) were brought to bear collectively to demonstrate their cumulative effect. According to variables in the cumulative strain model, long-term frustrations (chronic strains) experienced early in life or in adolescence—at home and/or at school—lead to social isolation; and the resultant lack of pro-social support systems (uncontrolled strain) in turn allows a short-term negative event (acute strain), be it real or imagined, to be particularly devastating. As such, the acute strain initiates a planning stage, wherein a mass killing is fantasized about as a masculine solution to regain lost feelings of control; and actions are taken to ensure the fantasy can become reality. The planning process concludes in a massacre facilitated by weapons that enable large body counts in schoolrooms and on campuses, where students are closely packed together and therefore convenient to kill in large numbers. When Bonanno and Levenson (2014) examined the life history of Adam Lanza, the perpetrator of the 2012 Sandy Hook Elementary School massacre, they concluded that "[a]lthough there may not be a clear-cut concrete explanation for why Adam Lanza committed a school shooting, at present, analysis of the evidence gathered seems to fit within Levin and Madfis's (2009) cumulative strain model and offer possible explanations" (p. 8). Likewise, Madfis and Levin (2013) discovered that, despite important international variations, the cumulative strain model applied remarkably well to international incidents of multiple-victim school shootings.

Beyond broad theoretical arguments, another clear indicator that school rampages serve a significant purpose for offenders is the profound level of detail involved in the planning of these events. As O'Toole (2000) points out, the planning involved in carrying out a school rampage is often a lengthy process. According to Vossekuil et al. (2002), most school rampage shooters create a plan at least two days before initiating their attack on students and/or teachers. Many of them develop and fantasize about their plots for weeks or even months prior to carrying them out (Fox & Levin, 1994; Madfis & Levin, 2013; Newman et al., 2004; Verlinden, Hersen, & Thomas, 2000; Vossekuil et al. ,2002). The Columbine killers, Eric Harris and Dylan Klebold, spent more than a year extensively preparing their attack (Larkin, 2007). In addition, among many of the cases of thwarted attacks studied by Madfis (2014a), evidence of planning a school rampage was often extensive. In this study, Madfis discusses myriad physical and digital evidence collected by police and/or school authorities to indicate extensive planning, such as the presence of hit lists and even "do not kill" lists, suicide notes, maps of the school with attack plans drawn on them, daily planners and journals describing the desired targets, methods, and outcomes, supply shopping lists, discussions about the plots on social media websites, and internet searches relating to research on how to execute an attack (such as for details about previous rampage shootings, attaining firearms, or building bombs). Plots were comprised of details such as who was to be purposely targeted and/

or saved, what locations were to be attacked in what order, and when the attacks were to take place. In addition to choosing a specific date for the attack, some students also designed plans for what was to take place in what order on the day itself.

While it is quite popular to depict mass shootings as the result of individuals simply "snapping" and committing violent onslaughts in a spur-of-the moment manner, this does not accurately describe the vast majority of mass murders, whether they occur on school grounds or elsewhere (Levin & Madfis, 2009). The extensive planning evident in most if not all of these cases indicates that rampage attacks unquestionably serve a purpose for the offenders committing them—whether it is about attaining vengeance, widespread infamy, a sense of masculine power, or a particularly cruel conclusion to long-term internal strife and interpersonal frustrations.

## School Rampages are not Patternless

School rampage perpetrators lack any single unifying profile (Vossekuil et al., 2002). However, recent research has gleaned discernable patterns among the individual characteristics (such as ethnic/racial and gender identity) of school rampage shooters and the social characteristics of the schools wherein they are more likely to occur. It is simply not the case that everyone in the population is equally likely to become a rampage shooter.

Both of the original school shooter profiles (Band & Harpold, 1999; McGee & DeBernardo, 1999) describe typical offenders as white males. In fact, mass murder, of which school rampage violence constitutes a subset, is the only form of homicide that is committed by non-Hispanic whites in numbers disproportionately high relative to their share of the population (Fox & Levin, 1998; Madfis 2014c). While it is certainly not the case that all school rampages have been committed by whites (for example, Oregon's Umpqua Community College shooter was bi-racial, the Red Lake Senior High School killer was Native American, the Virginia Tech shooter was Korean American, and the shooter at the Tasso da Silveira Municipal School was Brazilian), the majority of rampage killers have in fact been white. As a result, some researchers (Madfis, 2014c; Schiele & Stewart, 2001; Wise, 2001) have linked theoretically white racial identity and privilege to rampage killing.

Additionally, many researchers (Collier, 1998; Consalvo, 2003; Kimmel & Mahler, 2003; Klein, 2005; Mai & Alpert, 2000; Neroni, 2000; Schiele & Stewart, 2001) have observed that the vast majority of rampage school shooters have been male and asserted the role that dominant notions of masculinity play in the causing the phenomenon. In fact, there have been only five female school rampage shooting perpetrators in the history of the United States: Brenda Spencer, Laurie Dann, Jillian Spencer, Latina Williams, and Amy Bishop (though among these, only Brenda Spencer and Latina Williams ever attended the schools they attacked). Of the twenty-three students accused of being involved with planning an averted rampage attack at the eleven schools under investigation in Madfis' (2014a) study, only one was a female. While homicide in general is committed largely by males (Fox & Levin, 2014), nearly all school rampage offenders have been boys and men (Danner & Carmody, 2001; Kimmel & Mahler, 2003; Mai & Alpert, 2000). Accordingly, the role of masculine identity and gender socialization bear serious consideration. This may also relate to the fact that females have been heavily over- represented among the victims of school rampages (Klein, 2005; 2006).

School rampages are also patterned in terms of the types of communities and schools in which they most frequently occur. While the majority of American school gun violence in general occurs in urban areas, rampage school shootings typically occur at suburban and rural schools (Kimmel, 2008; Kimmel & Mahler, 2003; Madfis, 2014a) in less populated homogeneous communities located in ideologically conservative districts (Kimmel & Mahler, 2003; Newman et al., 2004). Much like their American counterparts, most international school rampages also occurred in small towns or villages with tightknit communities (Madfis & Levin, 2013). As a result, various scholars (Kimmel & Mahler, 2003; Madfis & Levin, 2013; Newman et al., 2004) have considered the role that the stultifying closeness and pressure to conform in small towns play in contributing to the phenomenon. Likewise, rampage attacks tend to take place in the context of particular social circumstances, such as when the school staff and student body are intolerant of differences (especially regarding gender nonconformity), when issues of bullying and marginalization are not addressed or taken seriously by teachers and administrators (Kimmel & Mahler, 2003; Levin & Madfis, 2009; Madfis & Levin, 2013; Newman et al., 2004; Vossekuil et al., 2002), and when schools foster punitive zero tolerance environments, which discourage students from coming forward to trusted adults when they hear crucial information about impending threats of violence (Madfis, 2014a, 2014b).

## School Rampages do not Represent Unqualified Deterioration

There has been a great deal of debate in the media and among academics recently about the extent to which mass and school shootings are becoming increasingly common (see, for example, Blair & Schweit, 2014; Everytown for Gun Safety, 2014; Follman, Pan, & Aronsen, 2013; Fox & DeLateur, 2014; Lott, 2014). Much of the disagreement here lies with how school shootings are defined and operationalized. Often it is the case that these numbers are politicized with gun control advocates favoring broad definitions so that the size of the problem is amplified and gun control opponents favoring far more specific criteria so as to minimize the extent of the problem. The broadest definition (Everytown for Gun Safety, 2014) includes all shooting incidents on school grounds regardless of whether shooters have any connection to the schools they attack, irrespective of how many people are killed or injured. Such an expansive operationalization typically includes suicides and gang-related violence, which are certainly consequential incidents worthy of quantification and concern, but they are qualitatively distinct in most ways from school rampage shootings.

Recent data analyzed by *Mother Jones* (Follman et al., 2013) conclude that mass killings more generally are on the rise; although Fox and DeLateur (2014) point out that this increase only holds for attacks in public places, as the growth disappears when domestic mass killings in private homes are included. However, schools are typically public locations, and distinct data analyzed by *Mother Jones* (Follman et al., 2013) and the FBI (Blair & Schweit, 2014) both conclude that school shootings have increased in recent years.

That said, and despite the manner in which extensive media coverage might suggest otherwise, rampage shootings at schools remain exceedingly rare. Compared to their homes and the streets, schools are the safest places for young people, and the risk of homicide for school-age youth is roughly 226 times greater outside of school than at school (National Center for School Safety, 2006). More generally in terms of probability, "only about 1 in 2,000,000 school-age youth will die from homicide or suicide at school each year" (Muschert

2007, p. 61) and "any given school can expect to experience a student homicide about once every 6,000 years" (Borum et al., 2010, p. 27). Accordingly, it is vital that parents, policy makers, and administrators do not exaggerate the frequency of school rampage attacks and overstate how likely these events are to occur. These rare but devastating events are far too frequently leveraged as justifications for profoundly enhancing punitive school discipline (such as zero tolerance policies with automatic suspensions, expulsions, and arrests) and amplifying security measures (such as metal detectors, surveillance cameras, and armed guards), which empirical research has not found to prevent rampage attacks but which do expand the school-to-prison pipeline wherein student misbehavior is punished more severely through the juvenile and criminal justice systems rather than in the educational system (Muschert & Madfis, 2013; Madfis, 2014a, 2014b; Madfis, 2016).

## When and How School Rampages are Random

Of course, school rampages are random in some ways. Many people who were not individually targeted but merely had the misfortune of being in the wrong school at the wrong time have certainly fallen victim to the random nature of rampage violence. In addition, the background "profiles" of school rampage offenders are surprisingly diverse and lacking in some discernable patterns. Thus, many of the identifiable criteria that one might hope to be able to utilize in order to provide helpful and predictive warnings signs lack reliability, and so, in this way, school rampage offenders remain troublingly random and unpredictable.

### Random Versus Targeted Victims

The extent to which certain individuals or groups have been targeted as potential victims constitutes a hotly contested debate, both internal and external to academia, about whether or not specific targets are victimized during a school rampage attack. Cullen (2009) argued that prior news accounts misreported the "myth" that the Columbine shooters specifically targeted minorities and jocks (see also Ogle, Eckman, & Leslie, 2003 on the media revisionism of this issue). Furthermore, some of the most groundbreaking and prolific scholars of school rampage (Muschert, 2007; Newman et al., 2004) explicitly define the phenomenon, at least in part, by victims being chosen randomly or symbolically.

However, Madfis' (2014a) study of averted threats of rampage school violence revealed that, in the majority of the cases in his sample, student plotters did in fact desire to target specific individuals or groups of people rather than, or in addition to, random victims and the school as a whole. In one incident, Madfis (2014a) found that:

> …the people the student planned to kill on the day of his attack were specifically chosen because they were individuals who he felt had slighted him in the past. For example, the sheet of paper found in his bedroom labeled "targets" contained the names of thirty students at the school, as well as the names of four additional students with "NK" (no kill) listed next to their names, and a distinct "Do Not Kill" section listing the names of another sixteen students. The student did tell police that his plan was not to kill strangers and only to kill those students who had been picking on him for years. There was also one girl in particular who he wanted to kill, and he had extensive written notes about her, such as where she lived and worked, what vehicle she drove, as well as exactly how he wanted to kill her by shooting her in the head…Further, he informed police that he added the names one by one, gradually over time. However, he also selected…"symbolic" targets…These included various cliques such as "Goths," "Punks,"

"Commies," "Hippies," "Preps," "Gays," "Ghetto Wiggers," and "Muslims" where asterisks were placed next to the names of certain students to indicate to which groups they belonged (p. 34).

Many of the other incidents explored in this study echo the same theme with would-be rampage killers specifically planning to execute disliked students and also taking additional steps to prevent harm coming to particular friends, though many also discussed attacking people more widely and randomly. This finding suggests that strict dichotomous distinctions between targeted and rampage violence are at least somewhat untenable.

### Genuine Patternlessness Among School Rampage Offender Profiles

While extant research has gleaned many discernable patterns among the individual characteristics of school rampage shooters and the types of communities in which they more typically occur, perpetrators lack any single unifying profile (Vossekuil et al., 2002). School rampage shooters are fairly diverse and, despite myriad efforts at locating clear and reliable warnings signs with predictive power, clear patterns simply do not exist in some areas. When one reads across the numerous occasionally contradictory studies which have investigated the previous problematic behaviors and social statuses of perpetrators of school violence, the literature can leave one with little more than a sense of random patternlessness the likes of which Best (1999) might find surprising and unsettling.

For example, many scholars have explored the previous problematic behaviors, whether inside or outside school, of rampage offenders in the hope of finding distinguishing features among their life histories. While one of the best predictors of violence in general is prior violent behavior (Campbell, 1991; Campbell, Breaux, Ewing, & Szumowski, 1986; Farrington, 1991; Moeller, 2001; Robins, 1966), the same cannot necessarily be said for perpetrators of school violence (Arluke & Madfis, 2014). In their study of school shooters, Verlinden and his colleagues (2000) found that nine out of the ten under investigation had some history of aggression and seven out of ten had a history of discipline problems. However, a report commissioned by The U.S. Secret Service and the U.S. Department of Education (Vossekuil et al., 2002) on incidents of targeted school violence found that just 13% of their sample of "attackers were known to have acted violently toward others at some point prior to the incident" (p. 22). Similarly, Vossekuil et al. (2002, pp. 20–22) found that only 27% had any prior arrest history, another 27% of the offending students had ever been suspended, only 10% had been expelled at some previous point in their lives, and 63% had never been or were rarely in trouble at school.

The other major area in which contemporary school rampage research has demonstrated less conclusive results than anticipated is with regard to the social status of school shooters. Being marginalized by and socially isolated from the rest of the school community are traits long associated with school shooter profiles and warning signs (Band & Harpold, 1999; Dwyer et al., 1998; McGee & DeBernardo, 1999), but subsequent empirical scholarship has provided mixed results. Some scholars (such as Langman, 2009a, 2009b; O'Toole, 2000; Vossekuil et al., 2002) have rejected the characterization of all rampage school shooters as "loners," while much case study research has found plentiful evidence of isolation and marginalization (for example, Lieberman, 2008; Madfis & Levin, 2013; Meloy, Hempel, Mohandie, Shiva, & Gray, 2001; Newman et al., 2004; Newman & Fox, 2009).

Similarly, affiliation with deviant subcultures has been thought to be linked with students who commit rampage attacks. This may be routed in much of the initial reaction to

Columbine when musician Marilyn Manson and the Gothic subculture (through associated attire like black trench coats) were blamed for inspiring the attack (Muzzatti, 2004; Ogle et al., 2003) and many scholars explored the role played by warning signs such as a "preoccupation with violent media/music" (Verlinden et al., 2000, p. 43) or "some interest in violence, through movies, video games, books, and other media" (Vossekuil et al., 2002, p. 22). Madfis (2014a) found that police and school staff took threats more seriously when the students making them demonstrated affinities for the music and clothing styles associated with certain subcultures such as Goths. Not only does the focus on these cultural preferences have the potential to marginalize a large segment of students who have done nothing wrong other than to subscribe to less traditional beliefs, values, and/or aesthetics, but it is a flawed guideline with little empirical basis. Numerous students who have attempted and completed school rampage shootings have dressed in a traditional manner. In fact, the official *Columbine Report* by the Jefferson County Sheriff's Office eventually debunked the notion that even Harris and Klebold "regularly cloak[ed] themselves in symbols associated with violence or the Goth culture; rather, they 'appeared outwardly normal, [sharing] their dark side only with each other'" (Ogle et al., 2003, p. 23). What's more, Madfis (2014a) found that one of the school rampage plotters he studied desired to deliberately target Goths as victims, and another rampage plot by popular student athletes on the wrestling team was taken less seriously by school officials, at least preliminarily, as a result of their clean cut appearance. Marysville-Pilchuck High School's school shooter was a popular member of the football team who had recently been named Homecoming Prince (Botelho, 2014).

Thus, successful and attempted school shooters are by no means monolithically Gothic loners, as they have come from a variety of school social statuses and cliques. In this sense, perpetrators can be thought of as at least somewhat random and lacking a clear pattern. Accordingly, simplistic stereotyping of school rampage offenders has the potential to be extremely harmful, especially when attempts are made to identify or target potential students based on broad criteria such as having few friends or identifying with youth subcultures. Risk assessments based upon the identification of characteristics, regardless of whether they are at the individual or group level, remain a contentious area of debate for scholars and practitioners alike. Although research has demonstrated that some descriptive traits have more reliable empirical backing than others, these distinctions are not widely understood. Consequently, problematic forms of risk prediction and assessment are still broadly considered in the decision making processes of school and police officials (Madfis, 2014a). In contrast, the threat assessment approach (Cornell & Sheras, 2006; O'Toole, 2000) evaluates how direct, detailed, developed, and actionable extant threats are in order to assess their seriousness. This approach not only helps to avoid unnecessarily targeting innocent students who simply share broad characteristics with some prior school rampage perpetrators (Cornell, 2013), but school and police officials who have actually averted rampage plots considered nuanced threat assessment criteria to be the most vital in prevention and the most useful in determining with certainty whether or not students actually intended to carry out their threats (Madfis, 2014a).

## Conclusion

All three of Best's (1999) assertions of randomness may demonstrate how media present incidents of violent crime, but they often do not represent the reality. Crime is not patternless, as victimization and offending patterns vary substantially by gender, race/ethnicity, class, age, and numerous other criteria. The trope of randomness perpetuates the misleading notion that violence is equally likely to happen to anyone and similarly that anyone can equally become a perpetrator. The idea of random violence inaccurately depicts crime as pointless, though even the most seemingly irrational misdeeds typically have a purpose in the mind of the offender. Likewise, it is problematic and inaccurate for media to depict the problem of violence as always getting worse, with higher crime rates as society falls apart. These same problematic tropes apply to the specific problem of multiple-victim school attacks. By analyzing and synthesizing the diverse literature on this phenomenon, this article has revealed and clarified the ways in which school rampage violence is and is not random.

The random trope (i.e., the notion that school rampages are happening everywhere at any time in a pointless and patternless fashion where everyone is equally likely to become a victim or offender) distorts the meaning and magnitude of these horrendous crimes. If the motivations, patterns, and trends of school rampage violence are not only misunderstood but actively thought not to exist, then the task of prevention is made far more difficult. Therefore, it is vital that scholars, policy makers, law enforcement professionals, and educators not only inform themselves about the true face of school rampage but maintain a skeptical stance when media or any other source seeks to simplistically portray this social problem as one of sheer randomness.

## References

Aitken, S. C. (2001). Schoolyard shootings: Racism, sexism and moral panics over teen violence. *Antipode, 33*(4), 594–600.

Altheide, D. L. (2009). The columbine shootings and the discourse of fear. *American Behavioral Scientist, 52*(10), 1354–1370.

Arluke, A., & Madfis, E. (2014). Animal abuse as a warning sign of school massacres: A critique and refinement. *Homicide Studies, 18*(1), 7–22.

Aronson, E. (2004). How the columbine high school tragedy could have been prevented. *Journal of Individual Psychology, 60*, 355–60.

Band, S. R., & Harpold, J. A. (1999). School violence: Lessons learned. *FBI Law Enforcement Bulletin, 68*, 9–16.

Best, J. (1999). *Random violence: How we talk about new crimes and new victims.* Berkeley, CA: University of California Press.

Best, J. (2002). Monster hype. *Education Next. 2*, 51–55.

Blair, J. P, & Schweit, K. W. (2014). *A Study of active shooter incidents, 2000–2013.* Texas State University and Federal Bureau of Investigation, U.S. Department of Justice, Washington D.C.

Bonanno, C., & Levenson, R. (2014). School shooters: History, current theoretical and empirical findings, and strategies for prevention. *SAGE Open*, 1–11.

Borum, R., Cornell, D., Modzeleski, W., & Jimerson, S. (2010). What can be done about school shootings?: A review of the evidence. *Educational Researcher*, 39(1), 27–37.

Botelho, G. (2014, October 24). Jaylen Fryberg: From homecoming prince to school killer. Retrieved February 28, 2016, from http://www.cnn.com/2014/10/24/us/washington-school-shooter/

Burgess, A., Garbarino, C., & Carlson, M. (2006). Pathological teasing and bullying turned deadly: Shooters and suicide. *Victims & Offenders*, 1, 1–13.

Burns, R., & Crawford, C. (1999). School shootings, the media, and public fear: Ingredients for a moral panic. *Crime, Law & Social Change*, 32, 147–168.

Campbell, S. B. (1991). Longitudinal studies of active and aggressive preschoolers: Individual differences in early behavior and in outcome. In D. Cicchetti & S. L. Toth (Eds.), *Internalizing and externalizing expressions of dysfunction: Volume 2 (Rochester Symposium on Developmental Psychopathology)* (pp. 57–90). Hillsdale, NJ: Lawrence Erlbaum.

Campbell, S. B., Breaux, A. M., Ewing, L. J., & Szumowski, E. K. (1986). Correlates and predictors of hyperactivity and aggression: A longitudinal study of parent-referred problem preschoolers. *Journal of Abnormal Child Psychology*, 14, 217–234.

Cohen, S. (2011). *Folk devils and moral panics: The creation of the mods and rockers*. New York: Routledge.

Collier, R. (1998). *Masculinities, Crime, and Criminology: Men, Heterosexuality, and the Criminal(ised) Other*. Thousand Oaks, CA: Sage.

Conklin, J. (2002). *Why crime rates fell*. Upper Saddle River, NJ: Prentice Hall.

Consalvo, M. (2003). The Monsters Next Door: Media Constructions of Boys and Masculinity. *Feminist Media Studies*, 3(1), 27–45.

Cornell, D. G. (2013). The Virginia student threat assessment guidelines: An empirically supported violence prevention strategy. In N. Böckler, W. Heitmeyer, P. Sitzer, & T. Seeger (Eds.), *School shootings: International research, case studies, and concepts for prevention* (pp. 379–400). New York, NY: Springer.

Cornell, D. G., & Sheras, P. L. (2006). *Guidelines for responding to student threats of violence*. Longmont, CO: Sopris West.

Cullen, D. (2009). *Columbine*. New York, NY: Twelve.

Danner, M., & Carmody, D. C. (2001). Missing gender in cases of infamous school violence: Investigating research and media explanations. *Justice Quarterly*, 18, 87–114.

Dwyer, K. P., Osher, D., & Warger, C. (1998). *Early Warning, Timely Response: A Guide to Safe Schools*. Washington, DC: U.S. Department of Education.

Everytown for Gun Safety. (2014, December 9). Analysis of school shootings. Retrieved February 25, 2016, from http://everytownresearch.org/reports/analysis-of-school-shootings/

Farrington, D. P. (1991). Childhood aggression and adult violence: Early precursors and later-life outcomes. In D. Pepler & K. Rubin (Eds.), *The development and treatment of childhood aggression* (pp. 5–29). Hillsdale, NJ: Lawrence Erlbaum.

Ferrell, J. (1997). Criminological verstehen: Inside the immediacy of crime. *Justice Quarterly*, 14(1), 3–23.

Follman, M., Pan, D., & Aronsen, G. (2013, February 27). A guide to mass shootings in America. *Mother Jones*. Retrieved February 25, 2016, from http://www.motherjones.com/special-reports/2012/12/gunsin-america-mass-shootings

Fox, J., & Savage, J. (2009). Mass Murder Goes to College: An Examination of Changes on College Campuses Following Virginia Tech. *American Behavioral Scientist*, 52(10), 1286–1308.

Fox, J. A., & Burstein, H. (2010). *Violence and security on campus: From preschool through college*. Santa Barbara, CA: Praeger.

Fox, J. A., & DeLateur, M. J. (2014). Mass shootings in America: Moving beyond Newtown. *Homicide Studies*, 18(1), 125–145.

Fox, J. A., & Levin, J. (1994). *Overkill: Mass Murder and Serial Killing Exposed*. New York: Plenum Press.

Fox, J. A, & Levin, J. (1998). Multiple homicide: Patterns of serial and mass murder. *Crime and Justice, 23*, 407–455.

Fox, J. A., & Levin, J. (2014). *Extreme killing: Understanding serial and mass murder.* Thousand Oaks, CA: Sage.

Fox, J. A., Levin, J., & Quinet, K. (2012). *The will to kill: Making sense of senseless murder* (4th ed.). Upper Saddle River, NJ: Pearson.

Glassner, B. (2010). *The culture of fear: Why Americans are afraid of the wrong things* (10h anniversary ed.). New York, NY: Basic Books.

Haider-Markel, D., & Joslyn, M. (2001). Gun Policy, Opinion, Tragedy, and Blame Attribution: The Conditional Influence of Issue Frames. *Journal of Politics, 63*, 520–43.

Henry, S. (2009). School violence beyond columbine: A complex problem in need of an interdisciplinary analysis. *American Behavioral Scientist, 52*(9), 1246–1265.

Hong, J. S., Cho, H., Allen-Meares, P., & Espelage, D. (2011). The social ecology of the Columbine high school shootings. *Children and Youth Services Review, 33*, 861–868.

James, S. D. (2009, April 13). Columbine Shootings 10 Years Later: Students, Teacher Still Haunted by Post-Traumatic Stress. ABC News. Retrieved June 15, 2016, from http://abcnews.go.com/Health/story?id=7300782

Killingbeck, D. (2001). The role of television news in the construction of school violence as a "Moral Panic." *Journal of Criminal Justice and Popular Culture, 8*(3), 186–202.

Kimmel, M. (2008). Profiling school shooters and shooters' schools: The cultural contexts of aggrieved entitlement and restorative masculinity. In B. Agger, & D. Luke (Eds.), *There is a gunman on campus: Tragedy and terror at Virginia Tech* (pp. 65–78). Lanham, MD: Rowman and Littlefield.

Kimmel, M., & Mahler, M. (2003). Adolescent masculinity, homophobia, and violence: Random school shootings, 1982–2001. *American Behavioral Scientist, 46*, 1439–1458.

Klein, J. (2005). Teaching her a lesson: Media misses boys' rage relating to girls in school shootings. *Crime, Media, Culture, 1*(1), 90–97.

Klein, J. (2006). An invisible problem: Everyday violence against girls in schools. *Theoretical Criminology, 10*(2), 147–177.

Klein, J. (2012). *The bully society: School shootings and the crisis of bullying in american schools.* New York, NY: NYU Press.

Langman, P. (2009a). *Why kids kill: Inside the minds of school shooters.* New York, NY: Palgrave Macmillan.

Langman, P. (2009b). Rampage school shooters: A typology. *Aggression and Violent Behavior, 14*(1), 79–86.

Lanier, M., Stuart, H., & Desire, A. (2015). *Essential criminology* (4th ed.). Boulder, CO: Westview.

Lankford, A. (2016). Fame-seeking rampage shooters: Initial findings and empirical predictions. *Aggression and Violent Behavior, 27*(1), 122–129.

Larkin, R. W. (2007). *Comprehending Columbine.* Philadelphia, PA: Temple University Press.

Larkin, R. W. (2009). The Columbine legacy: Rampage shootings as political acts. *American Behavioral Scientist, 52*(9), 1309–1326.

Lawrence, R. (2007). *School crime and juvenile justice.* New York, NY: Oxford University Press.

Lawrence, R. G., & Birkland, T. (2004). Guns, Hollywood, and school safety: Defining the school-shooting problem across the public arenas. *Social Science Quarterly, 85*, 1193–1207.

Leary, Mark R., Kowalski, R., Smith, L., & Phillips, S. (2003). Teasing, rejection, and violence: Case studies of the school shootings. *Aggressive Behavior, 29*, 202–214.

Levin, J., & Madfis, E. (2009). Mass murder at school and cumulative strain: A sequential model. *American Behavioral Scientist, 52*(9), 1227–1245.

Lickel, B., Schmader, T., & Hamilton, D. (2003). A Case of Collective Responsibility: Who Else Was to Blame for the Columbine High School Shootings? *Personality & Social Psychology Bulletin, 29*, 194–204.

Lieberman, J. A. (2008). *School shootings: What every parent and educator needs to know to protect our children.* New York, NY: Citadel Press.

Lott, J. (2014, February 17). Bloomberg's latest stats on school gun violence ignore reality. Retrieved February 23, 2016, from http://www.foxnews.com/opinion/2014/02/17/bloomberg-latest-stats-on-school-gun-violence-ignore-reality.html

Madfis, E. (2014a). *The risk of school rampage: Assessing and preventing threats of school violence.* New York, NY: Palgrave Macmillan.

Madfis, E. (2014b). Averting school rampage: Student intervention amid a persistent code of silence. *Youth Violence and Juvenile Justice, 12*(3), 229–249.

Madfis, E. (2014c). Triple entitlement and homicidal anger: An exploration of the intersectional identities of american mass murderers. *Men and Masculinities, 17*(1), 67–86.

Madfis, E. (2016). "It's better to overreact": School officials' fear and perceived risk of rampage attacks and the criminalization of American public schools." *Critical Criminology, 24*(1), 39–55.

Madfis, E., & Levin, J. (2013). School rampage in international perspective: The salience of cumulative strain theory. In N. Böckler, W. Heitmeyer, P. Sitzer, & T. Seeger (Eds.), *School shootings: International research, case studies, and concepts for prevention,* (pp. 79–104). New York, NY: Springer.

Mai, R., & Alpert, J. (2000). Separation and socialization: A feminist analysis of the school shootings at Columbine. *Journal for the Psychoanalysis of Culture and Society, 5,* 264–275.

McGee, J. P., & DeBernardo, C. (1999). The classroom avenger: A behavioral profile of school based shootings. *The Forensic Examiner, 8,* 16–18.

Meloy, J. R., Hempel, A., Mohandie, K., Shiva, A., & Gray, B. T. (2001). Offender and offense characteristics of a nonrandom sample of adolescent mass murders. *Journal of the American Academy of Child and Adolescent Psychiatry, 40*(6), 719–728.

Moeller, T. G. (2001). Youth aggression and violence: A psychological approach. Mahwah, NJ: Lawrence Erlbaum.

Molinet, J. (2014, October 27). "Senseless tragedy": Second girl dies in Washington state high school shooting. Retrieved February 2, 2016, from http://www.nydailynews.com/news/crime/girl-dies-washington-state-high-school-shooting-article-1.1988349.

Muschert, G. W. (2007). Research in school shootings. *Sociology Compass, 1*(1), 60–80.

Muschert, G. W., & Madfis, E. (2013). Fear of school violence in the Post-Columbine Era. In G. W. Muschert, S. Henry, N. Bracy, & A. Peguero (Eds.) *Responding to school violence: Confronting the columbine effect* (13–34). Boulder, CO: Lynne Rienner.

Muschert, G. W., & Peguero, A. (2010). The columbine effect and school anti-violence policy. *Research in Social Problems and Public Policy, 17,* 117–148.

Muzzatti, S. L. (2004). Criminalising marginality and resistance: Marilyn manson, columbine, and cultural criminology. In J. Ferrell, K. Hayward, W. Morrison, & M. Presdee (Eds.), *Cultural Criminology Unleashed* (pp. 143–154). London, UK: Glasshouse Press.

National Center for School Safety. (2006). Serious violence crimes in schools. Youth Violence Project.

Neroni, H. (2000). The men of Columbine: Violence and masculinity in American culture and film. *Journal for the Psychoanalysis of Culture and Society, 5,* 256–263.

Newman, K., & Fox, C. (2009). Repeat tragedy: Rampage shootings in American high school and college settings, 2002-2008. *American Behavioral Scientist, 52,* 1286–1308.

Newman, K., Fox, C., Roth, W., Mehta, J., & Harding, D. (2004). *Rampage: The social roots of school shooters.* New York, NY: Perseus Books.

Ogle, J. P., Eckman, M., & Leslie, C. A. (2003). Appearance cues and the shootings at Columbine High: Construction of a social problem in the print media. *Sociological Inquiry, 73*(1), 1–27.

O'Toole, M. E. (2000). *The school shooter: A threat assessment perspective.* Quantico, VA: Critical Incident Response Group, National Center for the Analysis of Violent Crime, FBI Academy. Retrieved March 20, 2016, from http://www.fbi.gov/stats-services/publications/school-shooter

Pinker, S. (2007, March 18). A history of violence. *New Republic.* Retrieved February 23, 2016, from https://newrepublic.com/article/77728/history-violence

Robins, L. (1966). *Deviant children grown up: A sociological and psychiatric study of sociopathic personality.* Baltimore, MD: Williams & Wilkins.

Rocque, M. (2012). Exploring school rampage shootings: Research, theory, and policy. *The Social Science Journal, 49,* 304–313.

Schiele, J. H., & Stewart, R. (2001). When white boys kill: An Afrocentric analysis. *Journal of Human Behavior in the Social Environment, 4*(4), 253–273.

Schug, R., & Fradella, H. (2014). *Mental illness and crime.* Thousand Oaks, CA: Sage.

Schwarz, E., & Kowalski, J. (1991). Malignant memories: Posttraumatic stress disorder in children and adults following a school shooting. *Journal of the American Academy of Child and Adolescent Psychiatry, 30*, 937–944.

Solomon, A. (2014, March 17). The Reckoning: The father of the Sandy Hook killer searches for answers. *The New Yorker*. Retrieved February 2, 2016, from http://www.newyorker.com/magazine/2014/03/17/the-reckoning

Sommer, F., Leuschner, V., & Scheithauer, H. (2014). Bullying, romantic rejection, and conflicts with teachers: The crucial role of social dynamics in the development of school shootingsa systematic review. *International Journal of Developmental Science, 8*, 3–24.

Velasquez, J. (2015, October 1). Cuomo calls again for stricter gun control laws after Oregon shooting. Retrieved May 22, 2016, from http://www.capitalnewyork.com/article/albany/2015/10/8578494/cuomo-calls-again-stricter-gun-laws-after-oregon-shooting

Verlinden, S., Hersen, M., & Thomas, J. (2000). Risk factors in school shootings. *Clinical Psychology Review, 20*(1), 3–56.

Volokh, A. (2000). A brief guide to school-violence prevention. *Journal of Law and Family Studies, 2*(2), 99–152.

Vossekuil, B., Fein, R., Reddy, M., Borum, R., & Modzeleski, W. (2002). *The final report and findings of the safe school initiative: Implications for the prevention of school attacks in the United States*. Washington, DC: U.S. Secret Service and U.S. Department of Education.

Webber, J. A. (2003). *Failure to hold: The politics of school violence*. New York, NY: Rowman & Littlefield.

Weber, M. (1978). *Economy and society*. Berkeley, CA: University of California Press.

Wike, T. L., & Fraser, M. W. (2009). School shootings: Making sense of the senseless. *Aggression and Violent Behavior, 14*(3), 162–169.

Wise, T. (2001). School shootings and white denial. *Multicultural Perspectives, 3*(4), 3–4.

Wolfgang, B. (2012, December 14). Shooting revives past horror schoolhouse violence. Retrieved May 22, 2016, from http://www.washingtontimes.com/news/2012/dec/14/newtown-conn-school-shooting-dredges-bad-memories/?page=all

# A Case Study of Paternal Filicide-Suicide: Personality Disorder, Motives, and Victim Choice

F. Declercq, R. Meganck, and K. Audenaert

**ABSTRACT**

Although evidence with respect to its prevalence is mixed, it is clear that fathers perpetrate a serious proportion of filicide. There also seems to be a consensus that paternal filicide has attracted less research attention than its maternal counterpart and is therefore less well understood. National registries are a very rich source of data, but they generally provide limited information about the perpetrator as psychiatric, psychological and behavioral data are often lacking. This paper presents a fully documented case of a paternal filicide. Noteworthy is that two motives were present: spousal revenge as well as altruism. The choice of the victim was in line with emerging evidence indicating that children with disabilities in general and with autism in particular are frequent victims of filicide-suicide. Finally, a schizoid personality disorder was diagnosed. Although research is quite scarce on that matter, some research outcomes have showed an association between schizoid personality disorder and homicide and violence.

The killing of a child is experienced as repugnant to reason. Paradoxically, the most probable perpetrators of child murder showed to be (one of) the parents (Alder & Polk, 1996; 2001; Cavanagh, Dobash, & Dobash, 2007; Stanton & Simpson, 2002). Moreover, filicide seems to be a leading cause of child death in wealthy industrialized nations (for a review, see Stanton & Simpson, 2002). Initially, it seems that women were most often blamed and punished for these crimes (West, Hatters-Friedman, & Resnick, 2009). However, it is clear that fathers also perpetrate a sizable proportion of filicide. Some studies have found that mothers are more likely to be the perpetrators of filicide than fathers (Kauppi, Kumpulainen, Karkola, Vanamo, & Merikanto, 2010; Laporte, Poulin, Marleau, Roy, & Webanck, 2003), whereas others have found that fathers commit filicide as often or even more often than mothers (Bourget & Gagné, 2005; Fedorowycz, 2001; Léveillée, Marleau, & Dubé, 2007). In any case, there appears to be a consensus that paternal filicide has clearly attracted less research effort and is therefore less well understood than its maternal counterpart (Adinkrah, 2003; Bourget & Gagné, 2002; Lucas et al., 2002; Marleau, Poulin, Webanck, Roy, & Laporte, 1999; Putkonen et al., 2011). The present paper seeks to contribute to a more elaborate understanding of this phenomenon by means of a fine-grained analysis of the underlying dynamics of a case of paternal filicide in which the offender provided full consent to the research procedure allowing for multiple perspectives on the case.

Bourget and Bradford (1990) introduced paternal filicide as a construct, thereby recognizing the importance of gender as a category in and of itself. Empirical evidence concerning paternal filicide suggests that, contrary to maternal filicide, the victims of fathers are often older children. Also, paternal filicide offenders appear to be much more likely than their maternal counterparts to commit or attempt suicide afterwards (Hatters-Friedman, Horwitz, & Resnick, 2005; Léveillée et al., 2007; Vanamo, Kauppi, Karkola, Merikanto, & Räsänen, 2001), which is also the case in the present study.

However, some points are atypical in the present case. Unlike mothers, fathers seem more likely to kill more than one child and pull along their spouses in the killing [familicide] (Léveillée et al., 2007; West et al., 2009). Regarding the motive, fathers also are more likely to commit filicide as a means or a reprisal against their spouse when going through a conjugal separation (Alder & Polk, 2001; Léveillée et al., 2007; Wilson, Daly, & Daniele, 1995). Although revenge was one of the motives in the case discussed here, the offender did not kill nor did he attempt to kill his two other children or his spouse. Instead, he deliberately focused on his son. Moreover, two root causes seemed to be intertwined, altruism in addition to revenge. To our knowledge, the scientific literature does not mention the presence of more than one motive in filicide.

Although filicidal fathers are more often diagnosed with alcohol and drug abuse and/or dependence (Putkonen et al., 2011; West et al., 2009), the offender discussed here had no history of substance abuse nor was he intoxicated during the offence. According to research findings, paternal filicide would also frequently take place in a context of prior domestic violence (Bourget, Grace, & Whitehurst, 2007; Jaffe, Campbell, Olszowy, & Hamilton, 2014) and prior abuse would be an indicator of risk of filicide (Browne & Lynch, 1995; Vanamo et al., 2001; Wilczynski, 1997), particularly when the abuse is perpetrated by the father (Bourget & Gagné, 2002; Putkonen et al., 2011; Wilczynski, 1997). Yet, there was no history of domestic violence or of child abuse in the present case.

Several studies have also shown that a large proportion of filicidal fathers are unemployed, have below-average education levels and a low socio-economic status (Bourget et al., 2007); Hatters-Friedman et al., 2005; West et al., 2009). At odds with these findings, the offender discussed here was self-employed, had a higher education level and a quite elevated socio-economic status. It seems that he fits the profile of a subgroup of employed filicidal men, described by Putkonen et al. (2011), whose problems are not of a socio-economic nature, but who have difficulties within adult relationships and have suicidal tendencies as a consequence of exhaustion and desperation.

With regard to psychiatric disorders, psychosis in general and schizophrenia in particular showed to be relevant diagnoses with respect to (maternal as well as) paternal filicide (Bourget & Gagné, 2005; Laursen et al., 2011; Marleau, Roy, Laporte, Webanck, & Poulin, 1995; Resnick, 1969). Within the spectrum of schizophreniform disorder, the offender discussed here could be diagnosed as having a schizoid personality disorder. Even though this disorder does not seem to appear in scientific literature on paternal filicide, empirical evidence has nevertheless shown a relationship between schizoid personality disorder and homicide (Hiscoke, Langstrom, Ottosson, & Grann, 2003; Loza & Hanna, 2006; Pera & Dailliet, 2005) and other violent crimes (Gvion et al. 2014; Hernandez-Avila et al. 2000).

Last but not least, a minimal amount of research has been dedicated to the incidence of disabilities among victims of filicide-suicide. However some empirical evidence indicates that children with developmental disabilities are at a greater risk of maltreatment and abuse (Ammerman, Hersen, van Hasselt, Lubetsky, & Sieck, 1994; Sobsey, Randall, & Parilla, 1997). More specifically, Palermo (2003) notes that of more than 1,600 cases of homicide in which the victims had a developmental disability 5% were persons with autism. Finally, by means of newspaper reports of filicides that occurred in the United States between 1982 and 2010, Coorg and Tournay (2012) found that children with disabilities in general, and with autism in particular, were the most frequent victims of filicide-suicide. In line with this research, Shields, Rolf, Goolsby, and Hunsaker (2015) report a case study of paternal filicide involving a 13 year-old victim with mental retardation. The victim discussed in the present study was diagnosed with autism and suffered from a hereditary illness.

With respect to research on paternal filicide, national registries are a very rich source of data due to the large sample sizes. Yet, as Hatters-Friedman and Resnick (2011) remark, such databases generally provide limited information on the perpetrator. Clinical, behavioral and motivational data, as well as knowledge of the offender's subjective experience are often lacking. Also, as previously discussed, the literature provides a lot of information concerning the general characteristics of paternal filicide, yet insight into the complexity of underlying dynamics remains scarce. As several authors suggest, the interaction between the constituting variables would be the key to understanding the risk for filicide (Dolan, Guly, Woods, & Fullam, 2003; Putkonen et al., 2011). Although single case studies have the disadvantage that their findings cannot be directly extrapolated, they provide a detailed account of the complex interactions among factors that lead to such violent conducts. Therefore, they are a powerful resource for deepening understanding and refining theory (Flyvbjerg, 2006; Stiles, 2009). Moreover, the strongly contextualized results facilitate transferability to similar situations, which implies that, despite restrictions with respect to formal generalization, they do shed light on the broader phenomenon of paternal filicide (Polit & Beck, 2010; Stiles, 1993).

## Method

The offender was willing to cooperate with the research project on violent crimes and all of the official data and records on the offence were made available to the researchers of the present study. The first author received permission from the criminal justice authorities as well as from the offender to study the official records for scientific purposes. The latter also signed an informed consent stating that interviews, test results, and elements of the dossier could be used for this purpose, if kept anonymous. Furthermore, the offender was informed that the study would not affect his status as a detainee in any way and that he could stop participating in the study at any time. Therefore, the present case study is the result of the analysis of the full official record and of the clinical assessment of the perpetrator. The interviews were conducted by the first author and took place in the penitentiaries where the offender resided. For the first interview, the official record/collateral information was not consulted in advance. The offender talked freely about his case. For the following interviews, the collateral information was reviewed thoroughly beforehand, giving the assessor the ability to probe for additional information and to investigate inconsistencies or deceptions. No inconsistencies or deceptions were found between the interview and the collateral information, which contained a variety of official records, the reconstruction of the offence, the autopsy, the toxicological analysis reports of officials' interviews with family members, friends, managers, co-workers, former teachers, etc., as well as the results of medical and psychological assessments. With respect to our assessment an Axis- I and Axis II diagnoses based on of the Structured Clinical Interview for DSM-IV Axis I and II disorders (SCID) (First, Spitzer, Gibbon, & Williams, 1997; First, Spitzer, Gibbon, Williams, & Benjamin, 1997). Psychometric properties of the SCID-I and SCID-II have been investigated with various populations and have also proved to be good (e.g., Maffei et al., 1997; Martin, Pollock, Bukstein, & Lynch, 2000; Weertman, Arntz, Dreessen, van Velzen, & Vertommen, 2003).

### The Offence

On the day of the fatality, the offender took his three children—two girls and a boy—to his parents for lunch, as was customary. After lunch he went shopping with them and bought a birthday present for his daughter. After that, he brought his two daughters back to their grandparents and drove off with his 9-year-old son, telling everybody they were going to buy him his birthday-present, which they did.

After arrival at the house where the offender had been staying since his divorce, he gave his son sleeping pills, telling him they were candy. He wanted his son to be unconscious in order "to spare him suffering." Unlike most perpetrators, who commit the filicide at their home (Marleau et al., 1999), the offender took his son to the hired garage behind the house, because he wanted it to happen in a "neutral place." When the drugs started to work, they headed to the garage. By then his son was in a semi-conscious state. He laid him carefully down on the ground and strangulated him with his bare hands in a face-to-face position. The autopsy report was in agreement with the offender's statements regarding the modus operandi and the pre-mortem condition of the victim. Indeed, the neck of the victim showed bruises that were characteristic of mechanical suffocation and the intoxication results as well as the absence of defensive wounds on the victim's body suggested that he must have been unconscious or semi-conscious when being strangulated. The body of the victim was found lying on its back covered with plastic folium that was stocked in the garage. His father had closed his eyes. When probed on the folium, the father said he had covered him because he wanted to "pull a sort of blanket over him."

The violence mode seemed to have been of an instrumental nature as the killing was intentional, purposeful, and lacking an affective display (McEllistrem, 2004; Meloy, 2006). The place where the homicide was perpetrated was selected in advance and the modus operandi (sedatives and strangulation) premeditated. The offender reported no agitation, anger, or shouting, nor did he mention fatigue or exhaustion after the homicide. Instead, he stated that he interacted calmly and gently with his son until the end. The lack of affective arousal was also verified from elements of the autopsy-report, as no signs were found that the medication had been forced or were defensive wounds found on the body. The disposal of the body—covered with a sort of blanket and the child's glasses carefully put aside on a shelf— and the very little disorder at the crime scene also point in the direction of a minimal affective arousal.

Leaving the premises, the offender went home and sent an e-mail to his ex-wife with cc to some of her colleagues and significant others. The subject of the mail was "dooms day." Two files were attached: in the first one he explained that he had killed his son because of his wife's infidelities; the second one—addressed to his two daughters—was a farewell note signed "your beloved father." Examination of his personal computer revealed that he had been working on these e-mails for a couple of weeks. After sending them, he put two birthday cards in stamped envelopes and dropped them into a mailbox: one was addressed to his daughter and one to his deceased son. The card to his daughter appeared to contain a farewell message, wishing her strength after his and her brother's deaths. The card to his son read: "Oh, dear X (name of his son), we're rejoining Y (the name of his firstborn daughter that died from a hereditary illness at the age of two) together, wherever this might be." He then drove around town "like a zombie" (sic.) until late at night.

He did not commit suicide immediately because the place he had selected for that purpose was not yet deserted,—with strollers still around, he was afraid his attempt might be noticed and prevented. Having chosen to hang himself, he selected a propitious place in advance and also bought a solid rope and a book on knots in order to make no mistakes. He planned to hang himself from a bridge instead of a tree, since he thought there was always a risk that a branch might break. When he arrived at the selected place, he took a cocktail of medications, which were prescribed to him for his depression and his sleep-disturbances, to overcome his inhibitions about killing himself. Yet, mentally blurred and drowsy, he was no longer capable to tie the rope and he staggered towards the river with the intention of drowning himself instead. However, he fell, injured himself and lost consciousness. Passersby found him with hands and head covered in blood.

### Pre-Offence Pathology

Mood disorder and depression are often found with paternal filicide offenders, although to lesser degree than with maternal ones. Like many filicidal men, the offender suffered from depression as he went through a conjugal separation (Léveillée et al., 2007; Alder & Polk, 2001)—this had led to a suicide attempt by means of a medication overdose a couple of months before the filicide. The treating physician and the psychiatrist he consulted at the time noted that he was at the end of his tether because of conjugal stress. Mental overload and desperation have indeed been associated with filicide (Putkonen et al., 2011; Mugavin, 2008). Notable, however, is that the depression and the subsequent suicide attempt were not related to hopelessness or to the fear of losing his spouse, as is commonly the case (Marleau et al., 1999; West et al., 2009). Instead, they were due to incessant quarrels over custody and especially over the way of raising their impaired son. Both parents seemed equally convinced of being right and both seemed equally belligerent to that effect. As a matter of fact, the perpetrators wife also attempted suicide in the period preceding the filicide.

The victim suffered from the hereditary illness that had killed their firstborn daughter years ago at the age of two. With their son, the illness manifested itself as a slight retardation in the locomotion. Moreover, the victim had autism and its frequent corollary: intellectual and language impairment. His mother became a militant supporter of a community-driven project that aimed at including impaired children in regular education instead of referring them to special education. To that effect, a community-sponsored attendant was assigned to the child. The father found this attendance during and after school unnecessary and his ex-wife's behavior toward their son pampering and detrimental.

During this period of dysphoria, withdrawal and isolation, the offender's thinking became egocentric and he started ruminating about filicide and suicide. Growing desperate, he began to have the idea "to leave this rotten life together with my son." When he consulted a physician and a psychiatrist concerning his depressive disorder, he did not have the courage to talk about his filicidal and suicidal ideations. As he had already been admitted to a hospital because of his previous suicide attempt, he felt that yet another psychiatric hospitalization would not help matters.

Having never had homicidal ideations before—and because they conflicted with his attachment to his son,—they were first rejected. The file information was perfectly clear about the fact that his children loved him and that he, albeit in a mainly cognitive way, loved them back. For instance, before the divorce, his children sometimes playfully competed over who would sit next to him in the sofa. After the divorce, the children liked to stay with him. His daughters visited him of their own free will and the eldest even chose to live with him instead of with her mother. They also visited him in prison after the homicide. Concerning his son, though, there was also another side to his attachment. Although he loved him, the offender admitted that, in fact, he was not very happy with him. He did not like having a son who was "different" and impaired. Although he admitted being ambivalent towards his son, he nevertheless stressed that this would not have been a sufficient reason to kill him.

Thus, the homicidal thoughts first met resistance and for a while the offender searched for other solutions. Not finding one, the thought that he "had to do something for my son before it was too late" started to hound him more frequently and with more intensity. As his thinking became more egocentric and the dysphoria became unbearable, his children informed him that their mother was seeing other men, and some stayed overnight. His jealous rage fueled his homicidal and suicidal ideations and seemed to have precipitated the offence (see the Motives section).

### Post-Offence Pathology

The offender attempted a well-planned suicide following the homicide. During his pre-trial incarceration he made more attempts to take his life. He first tried to hang himself with a belt. In a second attempt he cut his wrists with the splinters of a glass lamp-holder. Finally, he took medication that he had been collecting over time (neuroleptics, sleeping pills and tranquilizers). The records state that, in the last attempt he could only be saved *in extremis*. Closely related to his suicide attempts, the record of the prison psychiatrist mentioned a clinical depression based on a pronounced "taedium vitae," obsessive preoccupation with death, sleeplessness, apathy, bradykinesia, and anhedonia. During several periods, the offender refused food for several days, avoided all forms of social contact and spoke only when spoken to and only if speaking was unavoidable. During the reconstruction of the crime, he was nervous and showed avoidance reactions when in the vicinity of the garage. When asked to situate the place where the body had been left, he suddenly pulled back and started crying, covering his eyes and turning his back to the officials. The official report of the reconstruction further stated that he was able to describe the offence, and he could acknowledge or correct the reconstruction performed by an officer of the law, but that he appeared to be emotionally unable to re-enact the offence himself. The file also mentions that during his pre-trial detention a guard unintentionally overheard the offender say to another detainee that "seeing and feeling my hands is a daily torment." Although the filicide was intentional, it nevertheless seemed that the offender had strong guilt feelings afterwards and considered death to be the only appropriated sentence.

## Motives

Resnick (1969) was the first to propose a classification of filicide, which is based on its motive. Altruistic filicide (1) is committed with the motive of relieving the child of real or, most often, imaginary suffering. Thus, the parent kills the child because it is perceived to be in the child's interest, which may be the result of psychotic or non-psychotic reasoning. This type of filicide usually involves the offending parent's suicide (or attempted suicide). Acute psychotic filicides (2) involve severely ill parents who kill their children while in a psychotic state. In these cases the child is killed with no rational motive. In unwanted filicide (3), the victim is born unwanted and is a burden to the uncertain and incapable parent. Accidental death or fatal maltreatment filicides (4) are unintentional, due to single or recurrent episodes of battering. Finally, in the cases of spouse revenge filicides (5), the parent kills the child as a means of exacting revenge upon the spouse or other parent. In the case discussed here, a double motive was discovered: spousal revenge on one hand and altruism on the other.

### *Spousal Revenge*

As is frequently the case with paternal filicide, the homicide happened in the wake of a conjugal separation. Being unable to cope with his jealousy and rage toward his former spouse, the offender regarded the death of the child as a way to hurt her (Adinkrah, 2003; Alder & Polk, 1996, 2001; Cooper & Eaves, 1996; Léveillée et al., 2007). In the present case, the already tense situation related to the manner of rearing their son reached a paroxysm as the offender's son and daughters started complaining that their mother received men at home and that one of them slept in her bed. This made the offender furiously jealous—from then on, he considered his ex-wife to be an "adulterous whore." Some weeks before the offence, he told his daughters he intended to do something their mother "would not like." As a matter of fact, he would "hurt her into the core of her heart,"—and from then on, "every time she would sleep with a man, she would be reminded of her dead son."

The reason why he chose to kill his son instead of (one of) his two daughters, seemed to be determined by several reasons. Having a privileged position with regard to his mother because of his disability, the offender thought his demise would hurt her most. Also, the offender was convinced that the monetary allowance and the constant presence of an attendant made it possible for his wife to lead a promiscuous lifestyle. Hence, by killing his son, the monetary allowance would be withdrawn and his ex-wife would have to work in order to make a living and care for their daughters. It was the offender's perception that this would limit her liberty *casu quo* her presumed debauchery.

The offender's jealous rage toward the alleged lover that stayed overnight was apparently unreasonably exaggerated, though, as the man was hemiplegic. When it was suggested during the interviews that this person's medical condition excluded sexual intercourse, the offender stated that, "even so, a man sleeping in the mother's bed wasn't decent for the children and was disrespectful to their father."

### *Altruism*

The offender was convinced that his wife's effusive preoccupation with their son's impairment and her support of the educational inclusion project would be detrimental to their son. With his and his son's death, both of them would be liberated from what he experienced as the mother's intrusive and overbearing interference. Also, the offender had long been preoccupied with what would become of his son when he reached adulthood. He thought of his child as a nice boy and he believed that his son would be far too good to survive in what the offender considered to be a dog-eat-dog world. He was convinced that, by killing him, he would in fact spare him from a cruel destiny: "He wouldn't have a future and would only get in trouble, anyway." As it is often the case with individuals with schizoaffective disorders, the offender manifested a generalized distrust towards others and regarded the world as a malevolent place. As an example, the offender could not make sense of the penitentiary personnel saying "good morning" when opening the cells for breakfast. In his opinion "a morning could never qualify as good in prison." Hence, he suspected the guards were saying it to "torment and mock the detainees."

The following illustrates the peculiar form of empathy—coined by Blair (2005) as cognitive empathy—which individuals on the schizophrenic spectrums have been shown to manifest. When asked why he did not kill his spouse instead of his son,—since he wanted to retaliate against her and he viewed his dead son as "an innocent means and casualty to that effect,"—the offender answered that if he would have done so, the situation would have been worse. Driven by a singular form of empathy, he stated that if the mother of his two daughters was dead and he was dead (or in prison), their daughters would be orphans. This, he reasoned, would even be worse than the current situation.

### Personality Disorder

### Schizoid Personality Disorder (SPD)

One of the significant diagnostic categories that have been associated with (maternal and) paternal filicide, is a schizoaffective disorder. The offender did not report—nor did the collateral information indicate—the presence of hallucinations, conceptual disorganization, or magical ideation. Thus, he mainly presented the core negative symptoms, which revolve around blunted affect and social withdrawal.

Already as a child, the offender was described as reclusive and withdrawn. It was conspicuous to his parents that, unlike his brother, he did not have close friends and preferred to stay alone in his room instead of playing outside with other children. His social withdrawal and taciturnity were so familiar to his parents that his mother used to call him "William the Silent," after William I, Prince of Orange (1533–1584). They also grew used to the fact that he would lie on his bed or on a couch for hours, staring at the wall, without saying a word. As has been observed with individuals with this disorder, stress exacerbates the social withdrawal. Under these conditions, he was reported to be egocentric, unapproachable, mute and stubbornly opposed to interference (American Psychiatric Association, 2013; Rector, Beck, & Stolar, 2005). During his pre-trial incarceration, the offender would not only withdraw socially and give no or only evasive responses (prison personnel reported that he hardly said a word during his first year of detainment), but he would also barricade his cell from the inside and refuse to eat for days. When asked about this condition during the interviews, the offender said that, when he could not cope with stress any longer, "I just pull my plug out." When asked what goes on in his mind in these situations, he answered: "nothing ... or zeroes and ones" (see the following).

As an adult, he was primarily preoccupied with his family and his job. His employers and colleagues described him as very competent, or the best in his domain. Yet, on the interpersonal level—with clients, colleagues or the management—he was described as business-like, aloof, and unsociable. Detached and cold, the offender reported that he was not bothered by other people's opinions.

Because they cannot understand and respond appropriately to social stimuli, individuals with SPD are known to try to make sense of reality via peculiar cognitions or algorithms, and they form emotional attachments with objects or animals instead of people. Their impaired capacity to "intuitively" decipher other behaviors often leads them to scientific or mechanical-like analysis and explanations (Esterberg, Goulding, & Walker, 2010; Stanghellini & Ballerini, 2011). Constantly searching for "how things work," the offender used to dismantle and rebuild toys and objects as a child, and radios, televisions and so on when growing older. As an adult, he spent most of his time at his computer and he built a successful career in the technology sector as a specialist in computer networks. When asked during the interviews what this specialty consisted of, the offender explained that, it came down to making "several agencies *talk to each other*" (sic.).

Brilliant in mathematics, he would progressively and exhaustively approach and try to understand reality through mathematical algorithms. One of his major ones consisted of "binary systems, which come down to combinations of zeroes and ones." He gave the following explanation: "There is no such thing as grey. There is only black (0) and white (1). Grey is just a constellation where the numbers of ones outweighs the numbers of zeroes. So, it might *look* grey, but, in reality, it is still a constellation of black and white." It is on that ground that he explains (among other issues) his adamant unwillingness to discern or make compromises. Indeed, just like the color grey, compromises are deceptive and not straightforward. In his opinion, there would be less "hypocrisy, misunderstandings, deception and doubts if everybody would think in the same binary way. Unfortunately, most of the people are merged in and deformed by the grey, non-binary mode." Making sense of the mental states or behaviors of others through binary systems, it seems that the offender was genuinely unable to understand his son's sometimes impulsive, inappropriate social and rigid autistic behavior. To him it appeared that his son "lived on another planet." Discussing the offence, he emphasized that, contrary to human behavior, mathematically-based computer systems are regarded as "intelligent and reliable." As the offender explained, the output of a computer is determined by the input: "a computer can only produce a stupid answer if the initial question is stupid." "Hence intelligent input ineluctably leads to intelligent output." Although he did his best to feed his son with what he considered to be intelligent input, the output was not as he expected. As has been observed with individuals with schizoid personality disorder, the offender saw the world as being out of line rather than himself not being attuned with the world around him (Esterberg et al., 2010).

### Schizoid Personality Disorder and Violence

Although research is quite limited on the matter, some outcomes have shown an association between schizoid personality disorder and instrumental homicide and violence. Investigating the relationship between various personality disorders and criminal behavior among 370 drug- and alcohol-dependent patients during a year, it appeared that—even more than the antisocial and the borderline ones—the schizoid personality disorder had the strongest association with violent offences. Contrary to the first personality disorders, though, the relationship between the schizoid personality disorder and substance use and criminal versatility (weapon offences, property-, drug- or alcohol-related offences, major traffic violations etc.) was absent (Hernandez-Avila et al., 2000). Addressing the question of whether schizoid personality is a forerunner of homicidal or suicidal behavior, Loza and Hanna (2006) discussed the case of a schizoid individual who made a first unsuccessful attempt to murder his spouse and who—later, after several years of marriage, did kill her. After serving a sentence and on his way to being released, he committed suicide. Except for the violence against his wife, he had no history of drug- or alcohol abuse, violence, incarceration, or mental hospitalization.

## Discussion

Contrary to research findings, the offender was never involved with the law and he had no history of violence, incarceration or psychiatric antecedents, apart from a short hospitalization with respect to a suicide attempt. Also, he was not unemployed, did not have a below-average education level, nor did he have a low socio-economic status. Finally and exceptionally, there were two motives involved in the filicide: revenge and altruism.

In line with research results, the filicide discussed here evolved around the interaction of prototypical factors such as spousal separation and rage, desperation and filicidal and suicidal ideations. However these variables interacted with two others ones that are not well documented but appeared to have played a crucial role in the filicide, namely the disability of the victim and the schizoid personality disorder of the offender.

As his son was "an innocent means and casualty to that effect [hurting his ex-wife]", it seems as though the revenge motive was the more powerful of the two. Yet, his son's disability evidently fueled the offender's revenge feelings and his morbid altruism and thus determined the choice of the victim. Indeed, the offender never envisaged killing one of his daughters or committing familicide. Thus, his son's disability was at the origin of the offender's second, altruistic motive. If emerging empirical evidence points in that direction, further research might help establish whether or not children with disabilities,—and more particularly with autism,—are at greater risk for (paternal) filicide. Indeed an impaired child is often a source of concern inducing stress and hopelessness and mothers of autistic children appear to have more parenting and psychological stress than mothers of developmentally delayed children without autism (Estes et al., 2009). Children with autism can have impulsive outbursts, and bonding with them is difficult (Palermo, 2003). When these difficulties manifest themselves in an already distressing context of spousal separation and its frequent correlates,—depression, suicide, anger and resentment toward the ex-partner,- it is conceivable that children with disabilities and/or autism are at risk.

Furthermore, the present case reflects a critical interplay between the victim's disability and the offender's personality disorder. Individuals with a schizoid personality disorder have difficulty deciphering social clues and are oblivious to the nuances and subtleties of social interactions. Viewing him as "coming from another planet", the offender clearly could not make sense of his son's autistic conducts. In addition, and as it is the case for the offender discussed here, individuals with this disorder have proven to be prone to paranoid episodes, developing major depressive disorders and behaving in extremely violent ways in response to stress. Drawing upon emerging findings concerning schizoid personality disorder and violence, further research might shed light on whether this disorder can be a risk factor for (paternal) filicide.

It should be noted that the differential diagnoses of a schizoid personality disorder can be difficult to establish. Indeed, social withdrawal and alienation can also be found, for instance, in avoidant or narcissistic personality disorders or they can be the corollary of a severe depression (American Psychiatric Association, 2013). In the present case, the schizoid personality disorder went unrecognized and the offender was declared able to stand trial.

As most cases of paternal filicide are preceded by ruminations on filicidal ideations, Bourget et al. (2007) have suggested carefully enquiring about such ideations when the risk factors mentioned above are present. Although uneasiness with the issue of filicidal thoughts may prevent clinicians from asking about them and potential offenders from mentioning, in such circumstances, professionals might perhaps take the risk of addressing them. Indeed, the filicidal ideations were already present when the offender consulted professionals. At that time, he considered disclosing them but finally did not because he was afraid of adverse consequences. The possibility exists that if the professionals had addressed the matter respectfully and delicately, the offender might have disclosed these thoughts. Research findings or clinical evidence on the effect of addressing this issue in a clinical context would be most welcome.

## Acknowledgment

We would like to thank W. Vanhout and I. Storme from the Federal Government Department and Dr. E. Van Hoofstat, and the Penitentiaries of Brughes and Hasselt.

## References

Adinkrah, M. (2003). Men who kill their own children: Paternal filicide incidents in contemporary Fiji. *Child Abuse and Neglect, 27,* 557–568.

Alder, C., & Polk, K. (1996). Masculinity and child homicide. *British Journal of Criminology, 36,* 396–411.

Alder, C., & Polk, K. (2001). *Child victims of homicide.* Cambridge, UK: Cambridge University Press.

American Psychiatric Association. (2013). *Diagnostic and statistical manual of mental disorders* (5th ed.). Arlington, VA: American Psychiatric Association.

Ammerman, R. T., Hersen, M., van Hasselt, V. B., Lubetsky, M. J., & Sieck, W. R. (1994). Maltreatment in psychiatrically hospitalized children and adolescents with developmental disabilities: Prevalence and correlates. *Journal of the American Academy of Child and Adolescent Psychiatry, 33,* 567–576.

Blair, R. (2005). Responding to the emotions of others: Dissociating forms of empathy through the study of typical and psychiatric populations. *Consciousness and Cognition, 14,* 689–718.

Bourget, D., & Bradford, J. (1990). Homicidal parents. *Canadian Journal of Psychiatry, 35,* 233–238.

Bourget, D., & Gagné, P. (2002). Maternal filicide in Québec. *Journal of the American Academy of Psychiatry and the Law, 30,* 345–51.

Bourget, D., & Gagné, P. (2005). Paternal filicide in Quebec. *Journal of the American Academy of Psychiatry and the Law, 33,* 354–360.

Bourget, D., Grace, J., & Whitehurst, L. (2007). A review of maternal and paternal filicide. *Journal of the American Academy of Psychiatry and the Law, 35*, 74–82.

Browne K., & Lynch M. (1995). The nature and extent of child homicide and fatal abuse. *Child Abuse Review, 4*, 309–316.

Cavanagh, K., Dobash, R. E., & Dobash, R. P. (2007). The murder of children by fathers in the context of child abuse. *Child Abuse & Neglect, 31*, 731–746.

Cooper, M., & Eaves, D. (1996). Suicide following homicide in the family. *Violence Victims, 11*, 99–112.

Coorg, R., & Tournay, A. (2012). Filicide-suicide involving children with disabilities. *Journal of Child Neurology, 28*, 6, 745–751.

Dolan, M., Guly, O., Woods, P., & Fullam, R. (2003). Child homicide. *Medicine, Science and the Law, 43*, 153–169.

Esterberg, M., Goulding, S., & Walker, E. (2010). Cluster A Personality Disorders: Schizotypal, Schizoid and Paranoid Personality Disorders in Childhood and Adolescence. *Journal of Psychopathology and Behavioral Assessment, 32*, 515–528.

Estes, A., Munson, J., Dawson, G., Koehler, E., Zhou, X. H., & Abbott, R. (2009). Parenting stress and psychological functioning among mothers of preschool children with autism and developmental delay. *Autism, 13*, 375–387.

Fedorowycz, O. (2001). L'homicide au Canada [Homicide in Canada]. *Juristat, 21*, 1–18.

First, M. B., Spitzer, R. L., Gibbon, M., & Williams, J. B. W. (1997). *Structured clinical interview for DSM-IV axis I disorders.* Amsterdam, The Netherlands: Harcourt Test.

First, M. B., Spitzer, R. L., Gibbon, M., Williams, J. B. W., & Benjamin, J. (1997). *Structured clinical interview for DSM-IV axis II personality disorders.* Amsterdam, The Netherlands: Harcourt Test.

Flyvbjerg, B. (2006). Five misunderstandings about case study research. *Qualitative Inquiry, 12*, 219–245.

Gvion, Y., Horresh, N., Levi-Belz, Y, Fischel, T., Treves, I., Weiser, M., David, H., Stein-Reizer, O., & Apter, A. (2014). Aggression-impulsivity, mental pain, and communication difficulties in medically serious and medically non-serious suicide attempters. *Comprehensive Psychiatry, 55*, 1, 40–50.

Hatters-Friedman, S., Horwitz, S. M., & Resnick, P. J. (2005). Child murder by mothers: A critical analysis of the current state of knowledge and a research agenda. *American Journal of Psychiatry, 162*, 1578–1587.

Hatters-Friedman, S., & Resnick, P. (2011). Parents that kill: Why do they do it ?*Journal of Clinical Psychiatry, 72*, 5, 587–588.

Hernandez-Avila, C., Burleson, J., Poling, J., Tennen, H., Rounsaville, B., & Kranzler, H. (2000). Personality and substance use disorders as predictors of criminality. *Comprehensive Psychiatry, 41*, 4, 276–283.

Hiscoke, U., Langstrom, N., Ottosson, H., & Grann, M. (2003). Self-reported personality traits and disorders (DSM-IV) and risk of criminal recidivism: A prospective study. *Journal of Personality Disorders, 17*, 4, 293–305.

Jaffe, P. G., Campbell, M., Olszowy, L., & Hamilton, L. H. A. (2014). Paternal filicide in the context of domestic Violence: Challenges in risk assessment and risk management for community and justice professionals. *Child Abuse Review, 23*, 142–153.

Kauppi, A., Kumpulainen, K., Karkola, K., Vanamo, T., & Merikanto, J. (2010). *Journal of the American Academy of Psychiatry and the Law, 38*, 229–238.

Laporte, L., Poulin, B., Marleau, J., Roy, R., & Webanck, T. (2003). Filicidal women: jail or psychiatric ward? *Canadian Journal of Psychiatry, 48*, 94–98.

Laursen, T., Munk-Olsen, T., Mortensen, P., Abel, K., Appleby, L., & Webb, R. (2011). Filicide in offspring of parents with severe psychiatric disorders: A population-based cohort study of child homicide. *Journal of Clinical Psychiatry, 72*, 698–703.

Léveillée, S., Marleau, J., & Dubé, M. (2007). Filicide: a comparison by sex and presence or absence of self-destructive behavior. *Journal of Family Violence, 22*, 287–295.

Loza, W., & Hanna, S. (2006). Is schizoid personality disorder a forerunner of homicidal or suicidal behavior? *International Journal of Offender Therapy and Comparative Criminology, 50*, 3, 338–343.

Lucas, D., Wezner, K., Milner, J., McCanne, T., Harris, I., Munroe-Posey, C., & Nelson, J. (2002). Victim, perpetrator, family and incident characteristics of infant and child homicide in the United States Air Force. *Child Abuse & Neglect, 26,* 167–186.

Maffei, C., Fossati, A., Agostoni, I., Barraco, A., Bagnato, M., Deborah, D., …. & Petrachi, M. (1997). Interrater reliability and internal consistency of the structural clinical interview for DSM-IV axis II personality disorders (SCID-II), Version 2.0. *Journal of Personality Disorders, 11,* 279–284.

Marleau J., Poulin B., Webanck T., Roy, R., & Laporte, L. (1999). Paternal filicide: a study of 10 men. *Canadian Journal of Psychiatry, 44,* 57–63.

Marleau, J., Roy R., Laporte L, Webanck, T., & Poulin, B. (1995). Homicide d'enfants commis par la mère. *Canadian Journal of Psychiatry, 40,* 142–149.

Martin, C. S., Pollock, N. K., Bukstein, O. G., & Lynch, K. G. (2000). Inter-rater reliability of the SCID alcohol and substance use disorder section among adolescents. *Drug and Alcohol Dependence, 59,* 173–176.

McEllistrem, J. E. (2004). Affective and predatory violence: A bimodal classification system of human aggression and violence. *Aggression and Violent Behavior, 10,* 1–30.

Meloy, J. R. (2006). Empirical basis and forensic application of affective and predatory violence. *Australian and New Zealand Journal of Psychiatry, 40,* 539–547.

Mugavin, M. (2008). Maternal filicide theoretical framework. *Journal of Forensic Nursing, 4,* 68–79.

Palermo, M. (2003) Preventing filicide in families with autistic children. *International Journal of Offender Therapy and Comparative Criminology, 47,* 1, 47–57

Pera, S., & Dailliet, A. (2005). Homicide by mentally ill: clinical and criminological analysis. *Encéphale—Revue de Psychiatrie Clinique, Biologique et Thérapeutique, 31,* 5, 539–549.

Polit, D. F., & Beck, T. C. (2010). Generalization in quantitative and qualitative research: myths and strategies. *International Journal of Nursing Studies, 47,* 1451–1458.

Putkonen, H., Amon, S., Eronen, M., Klier, M., Almiron, M., Cederwall, J., & Weizmann-Henelius, G. (2011). Gender differences in filicide offense characteristics—A comprehensive register-based study of child murder in two European countries. *Child Abuse and Neglect, 35,* 319–328.

Rector, N., Beck, A., & Stolar, N. (2005). The negative symptoms of schizophrenia: A cognitive perspective, *Canadian Journal of Psychiatry, 50,* 5, 247–257.

Resnick, P. (1969). Child murder by parents: A psychiatric review of filicide. *American Journal of Psychiatry, 126,* 325–334.

Shields, L., Rolf, C., Goolsby, M., & Hunsaker, J. (2015). Filicide-suicide: Case series and review of the literature. *American Journal of Forensic Medicine, 36,* 3, 210–215.

Sobsey, D., Randall, W., & Parilla, R. K. (1997). Gender differences in abused children with and without disabilities. *Child Abuse and Neglect, 21,* 707–720.

Stanghellini, G., & Ballerini, M. (2011). What is it like to be a person with schizophrenia in the social world? A first-person perspective study in schizophrenic dissociality—part 2: Methodological issues and empirical findings. *Psychopathology, 44,* 183–192.

Stanton, J., & Simpson, A. (2002). Filicide: A review, *International Journal of Law and Psychiatry, 25,* 1–14.

Stiles, W. B. (1993). Quality control in qualitative research. *Clinical Psychology Review, 13,* 593–618.

Stiles, W. B. (2009). Logical operations in theory-building case studies. *Pragmatic case studies in psychotherapy, 5,* 9–22. Retrieved from http://pcsp.libraries.rutgers.edu

Vanamo, T., Kauppi, A., Karkola, K., Merikanto, J, & Räsänen, E. (2001). Intrafamilial homicide in Finland 1970–1994: Incidence, causes of death and demographic characteristics. *Forensic Science International, 17,* 199–204.

Weertman, A., Arntz, A., Dreessen, L., van Velzen, C., & Vertommen, S. (2003). Short interval test-retest interrater reliability of the Structured Clinical Interview for DSM-IV personality disorders (SCID II). *Journal of Personality Disorders, 17,* 562–567.

West, S., Hatters-Friedman, S., & Resnick P. (2009). Fathers who kill their children: An analysis of the literature. *Journal of Forensic Sciences, 54,* 463–468.

Wilczynski, A. (1997). *Child homicide.* London, UK: Greenwich Medical Media.

Wilson, M., Daly, M., & Daniele, A. (1995). Familicide: The killing of spouse and children. *Aggressive Behavior, 21,* 275–291.

# Violence is Rare in Autism: When It Does Occur, Is It Sometimes Extreme?

C. S. Allely, P. Wilson, H. Minnis, L Thompson, E. Yaksic, and C. Gillberg

**ABSTRACT**

A small body of literature has suggested that, rather than being more likely to engage in offending or violent behavior, individuals with autism spectrum disorder (ASD) may actually have an increased risk of being the victim rather than the perpetrator of violence (Sobsey, Wells, Lucardie, & Mansell, 1995). There is no evidence that people with ASD are more violent than those without ASD (Im, 2016). There is nevertheless a small subgroup of individuals with ASD who exhibit violent offending behaviours and our previous work has suggested that other factors, such as adverse childhood experiences, might be important in this subgroup (Allely, Minnis, Thompson, Wilson, & Gillberg, 2014). Fitzgerald (2015) highlights that school shootings and mass killings are not uncommonly carried out by individuals with neurodevelopmental disorders, with frequent evidence of warning indicators. The aim of the present review is to investigate this in more detail using the 73 mass shooting events identified by Mother Jones (motherjones.com) in their database for potential ASD features. There are 73 mass shooting events but there are two events where there is a pair of shooters which meant that 75 mass shooter cases were investigated. This exercise tentatively suggests evidence of ASD in six of 75 included cases (8%) which is about eight times higher when compared to the prevalence of ASD found in the general population worldwide (motherjones.com). The 8% figure for individuals with ASD involved mass killings is a conservative estimate. In addition to the six cases which provide the 8% figure, there were 16 other cases with some indication of ASD. Crucially, ASD may influence, but does not cause, an individual to commit extreme violent acts such as a mass shooting episode.

In their recent editorial article published in Autism, Maras, Mulcahy, and Crane (2015) aimed to debunk the myth that autism spectrum disorders (ASDs) cause criminal behavior. They highlight the fact that press reports serve to generate a speculative association between ASDs and criminal behavior using the example of the headline "Recipe for a serial killer? Childhood abuse, autism and head injuries are more common in murderers" (taken from the UK's Daily Mail following research by Allely et al., 2014). In our previous review (Allely et al., 2014) we decided to explore ASD to address the rapidly increasing media and academic reporting of violent crime (which largely consists of case reports or surveys of criminal groups) committed by offenders with ASD. Such attention has served to generate a speculative association between ASDs and offending behavior (Allen et al., 2008; Mukaddes & Topcu, 2006; Murphy, 2010). We concluded that "a significant proportion of mass or serial killers may have had neurodevelopmental disorders such as autism spectrum disorder or head injury" (Allely et al., 2014, p. 288). As highlighted by Maras and colleagues (2015), we then discuss the limitations of our study. For instance, much of the information was culled from online sources. Crucially though, the majority of mass/serial killers with ASD who were included in our review also had experienced other psychosocial risk factors for criminal behavior (e.g., physical or sexual abuse), suggesting that it is usually a complex combination of neurodevelopmental and environmental factors that is associated with acts of extreme violence, rather than autism alone.

Some studies, including those of "mentally abnormal" offenders incarcerated in special hospitals, suggest that the prevalence of ASD may be greater than that of the general population (e.g., Scragg & Shah, 1994). Silva, Leong, and Ferrari (2004) proposed the presence of an association between ASD and serial homicidal behavior, which has also been put forward by others (e.g., Fitzgerald, 2001). However, despite media speculation, surveys suggest that individuals with ASDs may be no more likely than the general population to engage in violent crime, and in fact, may be less likely (Mouridsen, Rich, Isager, & Nedergaard, 2008; Woodbury-Smith, Clare, Holland, & Kearns, 2006).

Hippler, Viding, Klicpera, and Happé (2010) conducted a study of penal register data regarding Hans Asperger's original group of 177 patients, and found that the rate and nature of crimes committed by these individuals were no different from that of the general population. In case records spanning 22 years and 33 convictions, there were only three cases of bodily injury, one case of robbery and one case of violent and threatening behavior (Hippler et al., 2010). It is crucial that these important findings are stressed in any dissemination of research regarding neurodevelopmental conditions and violent crime in order to avoid stigmatizing an already vulnerable group. Importantly, rather than being more likely to engage in offending behavior or violent behavior, individuals with ASD have been found to be at higher risk of being the victim rather than the perpetrator. Indeed, findings by Sobsey and colleagues (1995) indicate that individuals with developmental disabilities are between four and 10 times more at risk of being a victim of crime. Other studies have indicated that this group may be more than 10 times as likely to be a victim of sexual assault and more than 12 times as likely to become a victim of robbery (Modell & Mak, 2008). The hypothesis "that a complex interplay between neurodevelopmental and environmental factors—particularly psychosocial adversity—can result in an individual being predisposed to develop into a serial killer" (Allely et al., 2014) came about in response to the research literature suggesting that there may be a complex relationship between pre-existing neurodevelopmental problems (including autism spectrum disorder [ASD] [moderators], environmental insults experienced during development, including head injury or childhood maltreatment [mediators]) and serial or mass killing. James Fallon (2013) highlighted this complex interaction which can predispose someone to become a killer (Fallon, 2013, Naik, 2009). Fallon argues that violent offenders are often "created" from the combination of three key factors: genetic predisposition; damage to certain brain areas; and exposure to extreme trauma and/or poor parental bonding in childhood. With regard to the genetic factors there is strong evidence that there is an association between genes and violent crime. Monoamine oxidase A (MAO-A), for example, is an enzyme whose levels are genetically determined and is involved in the metabolism of norepinephrine, serotonin, and dopamine. Heide and Solomon (2006) showed that men with low MAO-A activity are three times more likely to be convicted of a violent crime by the time they are 26 years old compared to men with high MAO-A activity. One longitudinal study, which included 539 male children from birth to adulthood, found that the association between low levels of MAO-A activity and violence is only found in those who had also experienced childhood maltreatment (Caspi et al., 2002). The maltreated children exhibiting high levels of MAO-A expression were less likely to develop antisocial problems compared to the maltreated children with low levels of MAO-A (Caspi et al., 2002). Additionally, looking at adult violent conviction, maltreated males with low levels of MAO-A were more likely to be convicted of a violent crime compared to the non-maltreated males with low levels of MAO-A. Moreover, in the males with high levels of MAO-A activity, maltreatment was not found to confer significant risk for violent conviction (Caspi et al., 2002).

### Mass Shootings: Definition

Public mass shootings, also referred to as "active shootings" or "rampage shootings," present an unusual type of homicide (Lankford, 2015). There is confusion surrounding the definition of mass shootings or mass murder (Fox & Levin, 2015). Traditionally, a four-fatality minimum has been used to determine which incidents are "mass" shootings or "mass" murder (Duwe, 2007; FBI, 2008; Fox & Levin, 1994, 2015; Lankford, 2015). Public mass shooters shoot random strangers or bystanders in public places (e.g., such as schools, workplaces, theatres, or public streets), not just specific targets (Newman, Fox, Roth, Mehta, & Harding, 2004). About 38% of mass shooters commit suicide 'by their own hand' and approximately 10% successfully commit "suicide by cop" (Kelly, 2010 as cited in Fox & Levin, 2003).

### Mass Shooters and Mental Illness

Perhaps unsurprisingly, research has identified mental health issues or suicidality as being among the potential contributory factors underlying public mass shooting (e.g., Ames, 2005; Duncan, 1995; Fox & Levin, 1994; Langman, 2009; Lankford & Hakim, 2011; Newman & Fox, 2009; O'Toole, 2000; Rugala, 2003; Vossekuil, Fein, Reddy, Borum, & Modzeleski, 2002). However, it is important to emphasize that mental health issues by themselves do not cause an individual to carry out a mass shooting. Most individuals with mental health issues are nonviolent (Metzl & MacLeish, 2013). Rather, mental health issues may exacerbate other problems that are present in the individual's life which makes it more difficult for them to deal with issues such as family problems, problems in work or school, or personal crises (e.g., Langman, 2009; Lankford & Hakim, 2011; Newman & Fox, 2009; Newman et al., 2004). As highlighted by Lankford (2015), in individuals with psychological problems (such as narcissism, depression, psychopathy, paranoia) their perceptions of the world around them can become easily distorted (Langman, 2009; Newman & Fox, 2009; Newman et al., 2004). For instance, these psychological problems can result in irrational and exaggerated perceptions of their own victimization, bullying, and persecution subsequently resulting in their targeting of individual(s) who they perceive symbolize their persecutors (Newman et al., 2004; Lankford, 2015).

There are two primary 'sources of strain' reported by mass shooters which precipitated their act of extreme violence and vengeance. First, blocked goal achievement (e.g., being expelled from school or fired from work) and second, negative social interactions (e.g., bullying by fellow students) (Ames, 2005; Duncan, 1995; Duwe, 2007; Fox & Levin, 1994; Langman, 2009; Lankford & Hakim, 2011; Levin & Madfis, 2009; Lieberman, 2006; Newman & Fox, 2009; Newman et al., 2004; O'Toole, 2000; Rugala, 2003; Vossekuil et al., 2002). Mass shooters typically isolate themselves socially, cutting themselves off from emotional support and have relatively little or no close relationships or intimate contact with others (Fox & Levin, 2003; Hempel & Richards, 1999; Aitken, Oosthuizen, Emsley, & Seedat, 2008; Mullen, 2004; Levin & Madfis, 2009; Bowers, Holmes, & Rhom, 2010). Mass shooters are frequently single or divorced (Hempel & Richards, 1999), with no family or friends that can influence their behavior in a positive way (Levin & Madfis, 2009; Bowers et al., 2010).

### Challenges of Conducting Research in this Area

There are challenges in conducting research in this area, given that the event rate is so very low that the usual epidemiological techniques are not useful so systematic reviews assume greater importance. In order to investigate this area using conventional research techniques such as cohort studies, it would have to involve millions of individuals in order to have any chance of including an individual who commits a mass shooting event which is beyond the capacity of any funding body. As suggested in our previous paper (Allely et al., 2014) it may be that an adaptation of the research techniques used for extremely rare but dangerous diseases may need to be employed to investigate mass shooting events. Collaborative strategies have been developed by The World Health Organisation and European Union in order to carry out research on rare diseases (e.g., http://www.who.int/bulletin/volumes/90/6/12-020612/en/index.html) and such strategies may be required to understand mass shootings with the aim of implementing timely and appropriate interventions to reduce the risk of such event occurring. Lastly, and as mentioned in our previous paper (Allely et al., 2014), more rigorous research and the development of an international database is urgently required in order that reviews like our previous one and the present one "have a stronger foundation on which to report" (Allely et al., 2014, pp. 297).

### Adapted "Path to Intended Violence" Model to Understand Mass Violence in Individuals With ASD

What we have described so far in a very small subgroup of individuals with ASD has recently been highlighted by Faccini (2016) in his theoretical paper where he applied two different models in order to attempt to understand the intended mass violence in the case of Adam Lanza. The three factors of autism-based deficits, psychopathology and deficient psychosocial development was adapted to include the "Path to Intended Violence," to understand the possible route to mass shooting in a very small subgroup of individuals with ASD. The "Path to Violence" model is considered to comprise six behavioral stages according to Calhoun and Weston (2003). These six behavioral steps or stages include: holding a grievance (as a result of, for example, a perceived sense of injustice, a threat or loss, a need for fame, or revenge), ideation (considering violence to be the only option, discussing one's thoughts with others, or modelling oneself after other assailants), research/planning (gathering information regarding one's target, or stalking the target), preparations (such as collating one's costume, weapon(s), equipment, transportation, or engaging in "final act" behaviors), breach (assessing levels of security, devising "sneaky or covert approach"), and attack (Faccini, 2010).

To demonstrate how integrating the two models (previously described) can be applied to explain the process which leads to a mass shooting occurrence, Faccini (2016) outlines the case of Adam Lanza as an example. Faccini (2016) describes how Lanza experienced a sense of a threatening world as a result of the existence of a number of co-occurring issues including: difficulties with sensory processing, contamination rituals and exaggerated fears. Lanza's arrival at the first stage of the path toward violence, namely, grievance, which his sense of a threatening world was "exacerbated by progressive losses." In the case of Lanza "the nexus of the two models occurred when autistic restricted interests in death and violence, combined with depression and suicidal ideation, progressed into a fascination and restricted interest in mass shootings and shooters." (Faccini, 2016, p. 1). Additionally, Lanza's fascination with weapons and mass murderers was also consistent with the second of six stages ('ideation') in the Path to Violence model which subsequently lead to the shooting in Newtown. According to Faccini (2016) this model "presents with substantial face validity when applied to the mass shooting" (p. 1).

### Present Study

In 2010 it was estimated that there were 52 million cases of ASDs, a prevalence of 7.6 per 1,000 or one in 132 persons (rounded up to 0.8%) (Baxter et al., 2015). A recent population based study (based on the Child and Adolescent Twin Study and national patient register in Sweden) comprising of 19 993 twins (190 with ASD) and all children ($n = 1,078,975$; 4,620 with ASD) born in Sweden between 1993 to 2002 found the prevalence of the autism symptom phenotype to be 0.95% (95% confidence interval 0.82% to 1.08%) (Lundström, Reichenberg, Anckarsäter, Lichtenstein, & Gillberg, 2015). There is a very small subgroup of individuals with ASD who exhibit violent offending behaviors (Fitzgerald, 2010). In his recently published paper, Fitzgerald (2015) highlights that school shootings and mass killings are not uncommonly carried out by individuals with neurodevelopmental disorders with frequent evidence of warning indicators, and provides case study examples: Adam Lanza, Eric Harris, Dylan Klebold, and Cho Seung-Hui. The aim of the present review is to investigate this in more detail using the 73 mass shooting events identified by Mother Jones in their database for potential ASD features. There are 73 mass shooting events but there are two events where there is a pair of shooters which meant that 75 mass shooters (cases) were investigated. Previous studies and media reporting looking at the factors involved in, for instance, High School Shootings (e.g., the Columbine High School Shootings), tend to focus on potential contributory factors such as video games, music, Goth subculture and movies and tend not to explore the perpetrators' internal factors including depression, psychopathy traits, and neurodevelopmental disorders such as ASD (Lawrence & Birkland, 2004; Ferguson, Coulson, & Barnett, 2011).

## Methods

### How the Mass Shooters Were Identified for Inclusion for Further Study in This Review

In order to avoid the potential biases inherent in selecting mass shooters ourselves, we examined all cases identified by Mother Jones in their mass shooter database comprising 73 events from 1982–2015. As mentioned above, there are two events where there is a pair of shooters which meant that 75 mass shooters (cases) were investigated. The mass shooters investigated in the present review were thus not selected by the current authors. The Mother Jones database includes information on the attackers' profiles, the types of weapons they used, and the number of victims they injured and killed. The 73 mass shooting events in the Mother Jones database focus specifically on public mass shootings in which the motive appeared to be indiscriminate killing. They adopted the following criteria in order to identify cases:

- The shooter took the lives of at least four people in accordance with the FBI criterion. An FBI crime classification report identifies an individual as a mass murderer—versus a spree killer or a serial killer—if he kills four or more people in a single incident (not including himself), typically in a single location. If the shooter died or was hurt from injuries sustained during the incident, he is included in the total victim count. (But they excluded many cases in which there were three fatalities and the shooter also died, per the aforementioned FBI criterion.)
- The killings were carried out by a lone shooter. (Except in the case of the Columbine massacre and the Westside Middle School killings both of which involved two shooters.)
- The shootings occurred in a public place. (Except in the case of a party on private property in Crandon, Wisconsin, and another in Seattle, where crowds of strangers had gathered.) Crimes primarily related to gang activity, armed robbery, or domestic violence in homes are not included.
- The database includes a few cases known as "spree killings"—cases in which the killings occurred in more than one location over a short period of time, that otherwise fit the aforementioned criteria (http://www.motherjones.com/politics/2012/07/mass-shootings-map).

Crimes of armed robbery, gang violence, acts of terrorism, or domestic violence in a home were excluded and cases in which the motive appeared to be indiscriminate mass murder were included.

### Database Searches

Searches on other databases (described as follows) were conducted on each of the names of the mass murderers contained in the Mother Jones database. The Mother Jones database was therefore adopted as an independent non author-selected sample of mass murderers for further investigation based on inclusion and exclusion described below. Internet-based bibliographic databases (PsycARTICLES Full Text, Ovid MEDLINE(R) without Revisions 1996 to Present with Daily Update, PsycEXTRA 1908 to January 25, 2016 and PsycINFO 1806 to January Week 3 2016) were searched in order to identify papers which examined mass shooters (those identified in the Mother Jones database) and ASD. Searches on all four databases were originally conducted on the 28th January 2016. A separate search was conducted on all the four databases above for each of the mass shooters. The searches were not limited in terms of date of publication. The search criteria were set to identify the search terms as "keywords" within the text rather than "Title." The reason for this was to be more inclusive than exclusive, therefore potentially minimizing the risk that a relevant paper is missed during the search. With regard to the search words entered into the databases, we used the two strands of search terms for each mass shooter and only changed the third strand of search terms which was the name of the mass shooter. For example:

First search criteria strand - ["mass shoot*" OR "mass murder*" OR "mass kill*" OR murder* OR homicide*] AND Second search criteria strand - ["asperger*" OR "ASD" OR "autism spectrum disorder*" OR autis*] AND Third search criteria strand - ["Chris Mercer" OR "Chris Harper Mercer"]

Note that (as in the aforementioned example) if the mass shooter had a surname then the full name was entered as well as the name with the middle name removed in the event that a paper did not refer to the mass shooter using their full name.

Across all the searches conducted on each of the 75 cases only five research papers were identified of which two were duplicates. The remaining three texts were reviewed in full for relevant information pertaining to any ASD traits in the mass shooter discussed in the paper. Only two of the three made any specific reference to ASD in relation to the mass shooters being reviewed.

### Google Scholar

In addition to these database searches, numerous permutations of ASD (as used in the database searches outlined above: e.g., "asperger*," "ASD," "autism spectrum disorder*") and mass shooting and the name of the mass shooters identified in the Mother Jones database were entered into Google Scholar and searched for articles which were not identified through the database searches, for instance, [ASD AND "Chris Harper Mercer"]; [autism AND "Chris Harper Mercer"]; [ASD AND "Chris Harper Mercer" AND "mass shooter"]. The literature identified in these searches covered a broad range including court transcripts and newspapers articles. These searches were conducted during December 2015 and not limited by year of publication.

## Results

### Findings from the 75 Mass Shooting Cases

Of the total 75 cases in the database, information was found for six cases that referred to diagnosis of an ASD by family and friends or there were strong suggestions of ASD made by family and friends (Chris Harper Mercer; Adam Lanza; James Holmes; Ian Stawicki; Seung-Hui Cho, and Dean Allen Mellberg).

See Table 1 for the list of the 22 mass shooter cases where there was either strong evidence of ASD or symptoms/indications of ASD. As a result, from the total sample of 75 mass shooters, there was strong evidence of ASD in 8%.

There were a further 16 cases (21% of the total sample) where there were some indications of ASD traits (Pedro Vargas; Andrew Engeldinger; Wade Michael Page; Jared Loughner; Nidal Malik Hasan; Jiverly Wong; Steven Kazmierczak; Kyle Aaron Huff; Jeffrey Weise; Terry Michael Ratzmann; Michael McDermott; Larry Gene Ashbrook; Eric Harris; Gang Lu; George Hennard and Dylan Klebold). However, this needs to be interpreted with extreme caution as they are only ASD potential traits and do not equate with a diagnosis. See Table 1 for details of the 22 cases in the Mother Jones database indicating either strong evidence of ASD diagnosis or symptoms/indications of ASD.

### Case Study: Adam Lanza

On the December, 14, 2012, 20-year-old Adam Lanza killed 26 people, 20 of them young children, inside Sandy Hook Elementary School in Newtown, Connecticut (Cohen-Almagor, 2014). Solomon (2014) learned from his conversations with Adam's father, Peter Lanza, that

**Table 1.** Details of the 22 cases in the mother jones database indicating strong evidence of ASD diagnosis or symptoms/indications of ASD.

| Mass Shooter Case | Autism Spectrum Disorder |
| --- | --- |
| 1 Chris Harper Mercer | Diagnosis of Asperger's syndrome |
| 2 Pedro Vargas | Tentative suggestions consistent with ASD symptomology |
| 3 Adam Lanza | Diagnosis of Asperger's syndrome |
| 4 Andrew Engeldinger | Tentative suggestions consistent with ASD symptomology |
| 5 Wade Michael Page | Tentative suggestions consistent with ASD symptomology |
| 6 James Holmes | Strong evidence suggesting Asperger's syndrome |
| 7 Ian Stawicki | Strong suggestions consistent with ASD symptomology |
| 8 Jared Loughner | Tentative suggestions consistent with ASD symptomology |
| 9 Nidal Malik Hasan | Tentative suggestions consistent with ASD symptomology |
| 10 Jiverly Wong | Tentative suggestions consistent with ASD symptomology |
| 11 Steven Kazmierczak | Tentative suggestions consistent with ASD symptomology |
| 12 Seung-Hui Cho | Strong evidence suggesting Asperger's syndrome |
| 13 Kyle Aaron Huff | Tentative suggestions consistent with ASD symptomology |
| 14 Jeffrey Weise | Tentative suggestions consistent with ASD symptomology |
| 15 Terry Michael Ratzmann | Tentative suggestions consistent with ASD symptomology |
| 16 Michael McDermott | Tentative suggestions consistent with ASD symptomology |
| 17 Larry Gene Ashbrook | Tentative suggestions consistent with ASD symptomology |
| 18 Eric Harris | Tentative suggestions consistent with ASD symptomology |
| 19 Dean Allen Mellberg | Diagnosed with ASD |
| 20 Gang Lu | Tentative suggestions consistent with ASD symptomology |
| 21 George Hennard | Tentative suggestions consistent with ASD symptomology |
| 22 Dylan Klebold | Tentative suggestions consistent with ASD symptomology |

his son exhibited poor eye contact, problems with social relationships, preservation of sameness, narrow interests, impaired communication skills, and sensory issues. These features are consistent with Asperger's Syndrome according to the Diagnostic and Statistical Manual of Mental Disorders, 4th Edition (DSM IV, American Psychiatric Association, 2000) (Fitzgerald, 2010, 2015). The final report which outlined the findings from the investigation into the shooting was published on November 25, 2013. It concluded that the case was closed and confirmed that Adam Lanza did not have an accomplice. The report also referred to Adam Lanza's familiarity with and access to both firearms and ammunition as well as his obsession with mass murders (Pilkington, 2013; BBC News, 2013). In an article published in The New York Times it was reported that law enforcement officials had stated that Lanza spent the majority of his time engaged in solitary activities in his basement. The article went on to report that law enforcement officials believed that Lanza "may have taken target practice in the basement" (Kleinfield, Rivera, & Kovaleski, 2013). The shooter's second floor bedroom windows (and also the second floor computer room) were taped over with black trash bags. In the two years prior to the shooting, Lanza had decided to cut off contact with both his father and brother. While living with his mother in the same house, there was a stage where he would only communicate with her via email. The investigation following the shooting also found a document on Lanza's computer about the inherent selfishness of women, entitled "Selfish" (Curry, 2013).

A 48-page summary of the official investigation into the tragedy in Newtown was published on the November 25, 2013 that provided new details regarding Lanza's behavior prior to committing one of the worst mass shootings in United States history (Sedensky, 2013). Before the shooting, Lanza took out the hard drive from his computer and smashed it, which made the recovery of data very difficult for the investigators (Reports: Lanza smashed computer hard drive, 2012). Investigation of the evidence revealed that Lanza had a preoccupation with mass shootings and a significant interest in firearms (Pilkington, 2013; Sandy

Hook massacre: Adam Lanza acted alone and had an obsession with mass killings, 2013). Lanza is also believed by police to have researched previous mass shooting events extensively, for example the 2011 Norway attacks and the 2006 West Nickel Mines School shooting at a one-room school in Nickel Mines, Pennsylvania. Videos relating to the Columbine High School massacre, other shootings (e.g., Northern Illinois University 2008 shooting) and two videos of suicide by gunshot were also found by police to have been downloaded by Lanza (Winter, Rappleye, Alba, & Dahlgren, 2013). The report also contained detail on one of the findings from the investigation, which was a spreadsheet chronologically recording and detailing the events of mass murders that Adam had compiled (Altimari, 2013; Chappell, 2013). Specifically, it was a seven-by-four-foot sized spreadsheet with detail on approximately 500 mass murderers including information on the body counts and the weapons used. Such is the level of detail that it is believed to have involved years of work and used as a "score sheet" (in terms of body counts of the mass shootings, etc.) by Lanza (Lupica, 2013; Gendreau, 2013). One anonymous law enforcement veteran stated that "It sounded like a doctoral thesis, that was the quality of the research" (Lupica, 2013). It has also been reported that Lanza was particularly fascinated by Norwegian mass murderer, Anders Behring Breivik, and is believed to have researched him significantly and may even have replicated some of Breivik's "techniques" as Lanza used the same first person shooter video games for training purposes. Breivik was also reported to have been fascinated by other mass murderers (Lysiak, 2013).

At the start of elementary school, Lanza received a diagnosis of sensory-integration disorder. Sensory-integration disorder is one of the features of ASD but by itself it has no official psychiatric status. Lanza's parents, Peter and Nancy Lanza, in 2005 took Adam (when he was 13 years old) to see Psychiatrist Paul J. Fox who gave a diagnosis of Asperger's syndrome (a category that the American Psychiatric Association has since subsumed into the broader diagnosis of ASD). While his parents considered it to be useful to receive this diagnosis, Adam failed to accept it (Solomon, 2014). Lanza was also found to have obsessive-compulsive disorder (OCD) and was referred in October 2006 for treatment for his conditions. He was prescribed Celexa (Citalopram, an antidepressant) and behavioral-based therapy (Schwarz & Ramilo, 2014). It is reported that Lanza engaged in multiple daily rituals, was unable to touch door knobs without a tissue (for example), repeated hand washing and obsessive levels of clothes changing (Sedensky, 2013). However, Lanza's mother Nancy had strong objections to both the therapy and medication and Adam stopped taking the medication and attending the treatment sessions after just four visits (Schwarz & Ramilo, 2014). Lanza received his diagnosis of Asperger's disorder in 2005 and it is also reported at this time that he was exhibiting marked social impairment and extreme anxiety. Additionally, he was reported to lack empathy and displayed significantly rigid thought processes. His interpretation of written and verbal material was very literal, one of the symptomatic features of ASD (Gillberg, 1991, Sedensky, 2013). The psychiatrist who diagnosed Lanza recommended home-schooling stating that any potential negative impact of isolation from peers was far outweighed by the adverse impact that attending a regular school would have. Taking this advice, from eighth grade onward, Nancy taught Adam the humanities and twice a week Peter would work with Adam on the science related subjects (Solomon, 2014). Adam's father, Peter Lanza, in an interview in 2013 said he suspected that his son, in addition to his other condition, might have also suffered from undiagnosed schizophrenia (Solomon, 2014; Goodwin, 2013).

During the time he attended regular school, Lanza experienced extreme anxiety and discomfort with changes, noise, and physical contact with other people. Lanza's significant level of anxiety, Asperger's syndrome, OCD difficulties and sensory issues all had a significant adverse impact on his ability to engage with the school curriculum and, ultimately, his school performance. Tutoring, desensitization (behavior therapies), and medication were recommended, all of which were refused by Lanza (Sedensky, 2013). In seventh grade, one of Lanza's teachers described him as quiet, barely speaking or wanting to get involved in any activities. Teachers also reported that his writing assignments were strongly indicative of someone obsessed with battles, destruction and war compared to peers of a similar age. The extent of the violent content in his writing was considered disturbing (Sedensky, 2013; Christoffersen, 2013). He was also not known to have developed any close friends throughout his time in school (Halbfinger, 2012).

Lanza's parents took him to Yale's Child Study Center for further diagnosis when he was fourteen years of age (in 2006). The psychiatrist who assessed Adam was Robert King who noted that Adam presented as a "pale, gaunt, awkward young adolescent standing rigidly with downcast gaze and declining to shake hands." Additionally he "had relatively little spontaneous speech but responded in a flat tone with little inflection and almost mechanical prosody," which is a common feature in many individuals with ASD (Solomon, 2014). King also noted symptoms of OCD which is a common co-morbidity in individuals with ASD. He refused to touch metal objects (such as doorknobs) and did not like his mother to touch them either due to fears of contamination. "Adam imposes many strictures, which are increasingly onerous for mother," King noted. "He disapproves if mother leans on anything in the house because it is 'improper.'… He is also intolerant if mother brushes by his chair and objected to her new high heel boots, because they were 'too loud.' … If mother walks in front of him in the kitchen, he would insist she redo it." (Solomon, 2014). It was during this year (his fourteenth year) that Adam developed his obsession with killing and engaged in activities such as the well-informed editing of entries on mass murderers on Wikipedia (Solomon, 2014). Lanza's mother consistently described her son as having Asperger's syndrome over the years and had purchased a variety of books on the subject of Asperger's syndrome. She referred to a number of Asperger's syndrome characteristics displayed in her son such as an inability to establish eye contact, a light sensitivity, and significant distress at being touched by another person (Sedensky, 2013).

## Discussion

Exploring the presence of ASD in the 75 mass shooters identified by Mother Jones revealed evidence of likely ASD in six cases (8%) which is about eight times higher when compared to the prevalence (of under 1%) found in the general population worldwide.

Crucially, the findings of this review are not advancing the notion that individuals with ASD are more likely to be mass shooters or commit serious crime. There may, however, be a small subgroup of individuals with ASD who are more likely to become serious offenders, a claim supported by Fitzgerald (2010). Fitzgerald suggested that Autistic Psychopathy (Hans Asperger's own term for the syndrome that he described in 1944) may underlie the motivation of some serial killers (Fitzgerald, 2010). He posited a new diagnosis "Criminal Autistic Psychopathy," a subcategory of Asperger's syndrome. This diagnosis would help clearly differentiate this subgroup from the general population of individuals with ASDs, whom are almost certainly less likely to become involved in violent or criminal behaviors. We suggest that appropriate and timely interventions should be developed and implemented specifically tailored for individuals with ASD who may be at increased risk. In order to identify which individuals may be at increased risk research is urgently required to investigate which clusters of risk factors are more predictive of a mass shooting episode. Some researchers suggest that one of the possible warning signs or red flags is an increase in the intensity of preoccupations in an individual with ASD, particularly if those preoccupations have a sinister (disturbing or violent) content. In the case of Adam Lanza, forensic records show that he did develop an increased preoccupation with mass murders which was intense (Solomon, 2014). Mass shooting episodes are rarely impulsive and are typically methodically well-planned over some time and executed. This pathway to violence is important for the development of threat assessment for this small sub group. In the weeks or even years (as in the case of Norwegian mass shooter, Anders Behring Breivik who was also considered to have Asperger's syndrome; Daily Mail Reporter, 2012) where the potential mass shooter's violent thoughts, behaviors, and fantasies escalate, provides a time where identification can be made and appropriate interventions could potentially be put in place (such as ensuring such individuals do not have access to firearms). This process is typically instigated by a perceived grievance (such as a sense of injustice, need for fame, or revenge) that goes unabated, subsequently leading to the development of thoughts about harming others who may represent the individual or group who led to the perceived grievance. Ultimately, this then leads to the planning of the event. In the case of Elliot Rodgers (who is not found in the Mother Jones mass shooter database and, according to his mother, was diagnosed as having high-functioning Asperger's syndrome but who never received a formal medical diagnosis, Duke, 2014) he was convinced that women were unfairly denying him sex and fantasized for months about a "day of retribution.." In May 2014, he killed six people and injured 14 others near Santa Barbara, California (Follman, 2015). Some of the evidence of the well-planned nature of Elliot Rodger's attack includes the "Retribution" video, which he posted on YouTube several hours before the shooting that covered in detail his belief of being unfairly denied sex by women and not being able to get a girlfriend in addition to other grievances (Rodger, 2014a). Prior to the mass shooting event, he sent numerous friends, family, his teachers and his therapist a 107,000-word 'manifesto' he had written entitled "My Twisted World" (Rodger, 2014b). In this autobiography, Rodger maps out his life from his earliest memories to his plans for what he called the "Day of Retribution." A welfare check was conducted on Elliot Rodger prior to the attack, but a gun check was not conducted nor was any of Elliot Rodger's disturbing blogs and video reviewed. More research is required to explore these early warning signs in order to increase our understanding and recognition of the potential importance of such warning signs (The Secret Life of Elliot Rodger Interview, 2014).

Research exploring the psychological factors underlying very violent and apparently senseless behaviors such as mass shooting indicate that mental health issues may exacerbate other problems that are present in the individual's life making it more challenging for them to cope with problems in their lives (e.g., Langman, 2009; Lankford & Hakim, 2011; Newman & Fox, 2009; Newman et al., 2004). Similarly, having a diagnosis of ASD may in some cases *further exacerbate* other problems, making it harder to cope. This is particularly important to examine in more detail in light of the vast literature exploring the common co-morbidities which frequently present in individuals with ASD, most notably, mood disorders such as depression and anxiety (e.g., Ghaziuddin, Ghaziuddin, & Greden, 2002; Hammond & Hoffman, 2014; Matson & Williams, 2014; Moss, Howlin, Savage, Bolton, & Rutter, 2015;

Bruggink, Huisman, Vuijk, Kraaij, & Garnefski, 2016), and behavioral disorders such as attention-deficit/hyperactivity disorder (ADHD) (e.g., Chen et al., 2015; Taylor, Charman, & Ronald, 2015; Antshel, Zhang-James, Wagner, Ledesma, & Faraone, 2016). Such comorbidities may further intensify an individual with ASD's impaired ability to cope with problems in his or her life. A recent longitudinal study involving 124 youths with a clinical diagnosis of ASD (mean age, 10.6 ± 3.3 years) found that early comorbid psychopathologies including: anxiety/depression, inattention, hyperactivity/impulsivity and oppositional behaviors may further impair later social adjustment (adaptive functioning) in youths with ASD and highlights the importance of early identification and appropriate intervention of these comorbid conditions (Chiang & Gau, 2016). In a recent study 50 adult males (mean age 30 years), diagnosed with Asperger's syndrome in childhood, were followed up prospectively for nearly two decades (13–26 years) (Gillberg, Helles, Billstedt, & Gillberg, 2016). Investigating the comorbid psychiatric and neurodevelopmental disorders in this group over this time, it was found that only three of the 50 men had never met criteria for an additional psychiatric/neurodevelopmental diagnosis and more than half had ongoing comorbidity (most commonly either ADHD or depression or both), highlighting the clinical importance of a full psychiatric/neurodevelopmental assessment (Gillberg et al., 2016).

In addition to the co-morbidities experienced by individuals with ASD described above, numerous studies have found that children and adolescents with ASD are at increased risk of experiencing bullying compared to their typically developing peers (e.g., Little, 2002; Wainscot et al., 2008; Carter, 2009; Maïano, Normand, Salvas, Moullec, & Aimé, 2015; Humphrey & Hebron, 2015). Studies have also found that children and adolescents with ASD are at higher risk of victimization from their peers compared to their typically developing counterparts (e.g., Cappadocia, Weiss, & Pepler, 2012). This increased risk of peer victimization in individuals with ASD is associated with their social communication and behavioral difficulties, which also have a negative effect (Cappadocia et al., 2012). Studies carried out on the impact of bullying on typically developing children suggest that they are more likely to display a variety of negative behaviors and to experience mental health issues (e.g., have poorer social and emotional adjustment, exhibit depressive symptoms, anxiety, and clinically significant social problems; Mitchell, Ybarra, & Finkelhor, 2007; Nansel, Overpeck, Haynie, Ruan, & Scheidt, 2003; Ybarra & Mitchell, 2004). Furthermore, children with ASD may be at increased risk for adverse childhood experiences (ACE, e.g., violence, divorce) as a result of the behavioral and emotional issues and financial/social/emotional stressors, which are related to their care, as well as possible genetic vulnerabilities of family members. However, research investigating ACEs in children with ASD is sparse (Kerns & Lee, 2015). Another study looking at 121 adults with ASD found that, compared to the adult control group, adults with ASD did not use fewer cognitive emotion regulation strategies. Instead they used more "Other-blame" and less "Positive reappraisal" strategies (Bruggink et al., 2016). This has particular relevance when you apply this finding to cases of mass shooters such as that of Elliot Rodger who blamed others for his unhappiness—specifically women who he felt rejected him. Lastly, a recent study carried out by Leno et al. (2015) based on a sample of 92 adolescents with ASD found that they exhibited high rates of callous-unemotional traits. Importantly, the higher rates of callous-unemotional traits were not found to be strongly associated with conduct problems unlike in the general population (Leno et al., 2015). This study's findings provide further support to the theory that ASD is rarely being associated with actual violence.

## Limitations

As pointed out by Fox and DeLateur (2014), it is important to consider the potential limitations of the Mother Jones mass shooter database as it does not include all mass shootings. Instead it identified the cases which were considered to be senseless, random, or at least public in nature (Fox & DeLateur, 2014). Another potential limitation with the review is relating to the database created by Mother Jones which had specific criteria for inclusion of a mass shooting case (e.g., the shooter had to have taken the lives of at least four people; the killings were perpetrated by a single shooter; the shootings occurred during a single incident and in a public place and the murders were not related to armed robbery or gang activity). The Mother Jones database also only contains cases of mass shootings that occurred in the United States, which is a limitation. Moreover, it is not clear whether this database, given the strict inclusion and exclusion criteria, has included all possible mass shooting events. For instance, the case of Elliot Rodger (which we covered in the Discussion section) is not included in the Mother Jones database.

However, as pointed out by Fox and DeLateur (2014) such inclusion criteria exclude cases of mass shootings involving family members, despite such cases sometimes involving significant body counts. Additionally, the criteria applied by the creators of the Mother Jones database have also been argued to have not been consistently applied (Fox, 2013). For instance, Mother Jones included the Columbine mass murder and the Westside Middle School massacre even though they were perpetrated by more than one individual. In response to the criticism levelled at the creation of the database, Mother Jones highlighted that there is a need for a more specific focus on "senseless" public shootings and the importance of investigating mass shootings irrespective of just the body counts (Follman et al., 2013). Lastly, Fox and DeLateur (2014) also argue by only including shootings, which were not related to armed robbery or gang activity is limiting. Our understanding of mass shootings can also be increased by widening the net and including all types of mass shootings (Fox & DeLateur, 2014).

## Future Directions

Maras et al. (2015) conclude in their recent editorial letter that more rigorous research in this area is needed. Skrapec's (2001) research highlights that there is a need to renew our commitment to empiricism in the current respective approaches to the research of mass murder and serial homicide which will take us a step further toward being able to more accurately describe and ultimately understand this extremely violent behavior (a view consistent with others such as Kraemer, Lord and Heilbrun (2004) and Culhane, Hilstad, Freng, and Gray (2011)). Large databases will aid our efforts to uncover potential linkages between environmental factors and genetic components. To our knowledge, the Radford/FGCU Serial Killer Database, which catalogues a sample of 4,274 atypical homicide offenders, is the only repository of its nature fully available to researchers, practitioners and law enforcement professionals. Information is derived from a variety of different sources including prison records, databases such as Westlaw UK, exonerations, media sources, true crime books, and the Internet (Aamodt, 2015). Furthermore, the Serial Homicide Expertise and Information Sharing Collaborative (SHEISC) brought together an interdisciplinary team to share rigorously collected serial homicide offender data with the Radford data collection effort (Boyne, 2014) forming the first ever international multiple homicide offender database because, as Hinch and Hepburn (1998) strongly argues, data should be accessible. Yaksic (2015) discusses how we can address the challenges and limitations of utilizing data to study serial homicide (serial homicide and mass shooting, etc.) and discusses the importance of the further development and sharing of information through databases such as the Serial Homicide Expertise and Information Sharing Collaborative and the Radford/FGCU Serial Killer Database Project.

### *Conclusion*

Despite mass shooting being of modest interest to law enforcement professionals due to the fact that such crimes have a high clearance rate (the perpetrators often commit suicide following the incident or are shot by police on scene) it remains of great importance to understand the possible stressors, traits and antecedents to these events in order to implement intervention and to prevent such episodes occurring.

Currently there are enormous gaps in our understanding of the mechanisms underlying the development of a mass shooter (Bowers et al., 2010). One of the primary reasons for this type of research still being in its infancy is the fact that conventional research techniques would struggle in attempting to address these gaps in our understanding. In order to investigate the developmental pathways to serious violent offending like mass shooting, cohort studies would have to involve millions of individuals to have any chance of including someone who ends up committing these kinds of crimes. This method is clearly beyond the capacity of any funding body and research techniques used for extremely rare but dangerous diseases may need to be adapted to accomplish this purpose. For example, the World Health Organisation and European Union have developed collaborative strategies to conduct research on rare diseases and similar technology may be required to understand—and hopefully prevent—serial and mass shootings. This may be the only way we will eventually be able to confidently determine the prevalence, etiological factors and developmental trajectories associated with mass shooting.

# References

Aamodt, M. G. (2015, November 23). *Serial killer statistics.* Retrieved February 24, 2016, from http://maamodt.asp.radford.edu/serialkillerinformationcenter/projectdescription.html

Aitken, L., Oosthuizen, P., Emsley, R., & Seedat, S. (2008). Mass murders: Implications for mental health professionals. *The International Journal of Psychiatry in Medicine, 38*(3), 261–269. doi:10.2190/PM.38.3.c

Allely, C. S., Minnis, H., Thompson, L., Wilson, P., & Gillberg, C. (2014). Neurodevelopmental and psychosocial risk factors in serial killers and mass murderers. *Aggression and Violent Behavior, 19*(3), 288–301. doi:10.1016/j.avb.2014.04.004

Allen, D., Evans, C., Hider, A., Hawkins, S., Peckett, H., & Morgan, H. (2008). Offending behaviour in adults with Asperger syndrome. *Journal of Autism and Developmental Disorders, 38*(4), 748–758. doi:10.1007/s10803-007-0442-9

Altimari, D. (2013). *Police release documents on newtown massacre.* Hartford Courant. December 27, 2013. Retrieved February 4, 2016, from http://articles.courant.com/2013-12-28/news/hc-sandy-hook-state-police-report-20131227_1_adam-lanza-nancy-lanza-yogananda-street

American Psychiatric Association. (2000). *Diagnostic and statistical manual of mental disorders.* (4th ed., text rev.). Washington, DC: Author.

Ames, M. (2005). *Going postal: From Reagan's workplaces to Clinton's Columbine and beyond.* Brooklyn. New York, NY: Soft Skull.

Antshel, K. M., Zhang-James, Y., Wagner, K., Ledesma, A., & Faraone, S. V. (2016). An update on the comorbidity of ASD and ADHD: A focus on clinical management. *Expert Review of Neurotherapeutics, 16*(3), 279–293. doi:10.1586/14737175.2016.1146591

Asperger, H. (1944–1991). Die "Autistischen Psychopathen". i.m Kindesalter, Archives fur Psychiatrie und Nervenkrankheitem 117, 67–136. Translated in U. Frith (Eds.), *Autism and Asperger's syndrome* (pp. 39–92). Cambridge University Press.

Asperger, H. (1991). "Autistic psychopathy" in childhood. In Frith, U. (Ed.), *Autism and Asperger Syndrome* (pp. 37–92). Cambridge, U.K.: Cambridge University Press.

Baxter, A. J., Brugha, T. S., Erskine, H. E., Scheurer, R. W., Vos, T., & Scott, J. G. (2015). The epidemiology and global burden of autism spectrum disorders. *Psychological Medicine, 45*(03), 601–613. doi:http://dx.doi.org/10.1017/S003329171400172X

BBC News. (2013). *BBC News. Newtown gunman Adam Lanza had 'obsession' with Columbine.* November 26, 2013. Retrieved February 4, 2016, from http://www.bbc.co.uk/news/world-us-canada-25097127

Boyne, E. S. (2014). Serial Homicide Collaborative Brings Research Data Together. (Fall/Winter 2014). Criminal Justice Update (CJ Update). *An online newsletter for criminal justice educators.* From Routledge and Anderson. Vol. 43, No. 1, page 2.

Bowers, T. G., Holmes, E. S., & Rhom, A. (2010). The nature of mass murder and autogenic massacre. *Journal of Police and Criminal Psychology, 25*(2), 59–66. doi:10.1007/s11896-009-9059-6

Bruggink, A., Huisman, S., Vuijk, R., Kraaij, V., & Garnefski, N. (2016). Cognitive emotion regulation, anxiety and depression in adults with autism spectrum disorder. *Research in Autism Spectrum Disorders, 22*, 34–44. doi:10.1016/j.rasd.2015.11.003

Calhoun, F. S., & Weston, S. W. (2003). *Contemporary threat management : A practical guide for identifying, assessing, and managing individuals of violent intent.* San Diego, CA.: Specialized Training Services.

Cappadocia, M. C., Weiss, J. A., & Pepler, D. (2012). Bullying experiences among children and youth with autism spectrum disorders. *Journal of Autism and Developmental Disorders, 42*(2), 266–277. doi:10.1007/s10803-011-1241-x

Carter, S. (2009). Bullying of students with Asperger Syndrome. *Issues in Comprehensive Pediatric Nursing, 32,* 145–154. doi:10.1080/01460860903062782

Caspi, A., McClay, J., Moffitt, T. E., Mill, J., Martin, J., Craig, I. W., Taylor, A., & Poulton, R. (2002). Role of genotype in the cycle of violence in maltreated children. *Science, 297*(5582), 851–854. doi:10.1126/science.1072290

Chappell, B. (November 25, 2013). *No motive in newtown report, but many details about Lanza.* NPR. Retrieved February 4, 2016, from http://www.npr.org/sections/thetwo-way/2013/11/25/247219204/no-motive-in-newtown-report-but-many-details-about-lanza

Chen, M. H., Wei, H. T., Chen, L. C., Su, T. P., Bai, Y. M., Hsu, J. W., & Chen, Y. S. (2015). Autistic spectrum disorder, attention deficit hyperactivity disorder, and psychiatric comorbidities: A nationwide study. *Research in Autism Spectrum Disorders, 10,* 1–6. doi:10.1016/j.rasd.2014.10.014

Chiang, H. L., & Gau, S. S. F. (2016). Comorbid psychiatric conditions as mediators to predict later social adjustment in youths with autism spectrum disorder. *Journal of Child Psychology and Psychiatry, 57*(1), 103–111. doi:10.1111/jcpp.12450

Christoffersen, J. (2013). Police file on Newtown yields chilling portrait". *The Washington Post.* Associated Press. December 27, 2013. Retrieved February, 2016, from https://www.washingtonpost.com/politics/police-file-on-newtown-yields-chilling-portrait-of-shooter-and-more-details-of-ram page/2013/12/27/2d09a548-6f4b-11e3-b405-7e360f7e9fd2_story.html

Cohen-Almagor, R. (2014). People do not just snap: Watching the electronic trails of potential murderers. *Journal of Civil and Legal Sciences, 3,* 113. doi:10.4172/2169-0170.1000113

Culhane, S. E., Hilstad, S. M., Freng, A., & Gray, M. J. (2011). Self-reported psychopathology in a convicted serial killer. *Journal of Investigative Psychology and Offender Profiling, 8*(1), 1–21. doi:10.1002/jip.129

Curry, C. (2013). *Sandy hook report: Inside gunman adam Lanza's bedroom";.* ABC News. November 25, 2013. Retrieved February 2016, from http://abcnews.go.com/US/sandy-hook-report-inside-gun man-adam-lanzas-bedroom/story?id=21009111

Daily Mail Reporter. (2012). *Mass killer Breivik may have rare forms of Aspergers and Tourette's syndromes, says Norway's leading psychiatrist.* Mail Online. Retrieved February 5, 2016, from http://www.dailymail.co.uk/news/article-2156530/Anders-Behring-Breivik-rare-forms-Aspergers-Tour ette-s-syndromes-says-Norways-leading-psychiatrist.html#ixzz3zJg6kmXL

Duke, A. (2014). *California killer's family struggled with money, court documents show.* CNN. Retrieved February 5, 2016, from http://edition.cnn.com/2014/05/27/justice/california-elliot-rodger-wealth/

Duncan, S. (1995). Death in the office: Workplace homicides. *FBI Law Enforcement Bulletin, 64*(4), 20–25.

Duwe, G. (2007). *Mass murder in the United States: A history.* Jefferson, NC: McFarland.

Faccini, L. (2010). The man who howled wolf: Diagnostic and treatment considerations for a person with ASD and impersonal repetitive fire, bomb and presidential threats. *American Journal of Forensic Psychiatry, 31*(4), 47.

Faccini, L. (2016). The application of the models of autism, psychopathology and deficient Eriksonian development and the path of intended violence to understand the Newtown shooting. *Archives of Forensic Psychology, 1*(3), 1–13.

Fallon, J. (2013). *The psychopath inside: A neuroscientist's personal journey into the dark side of the brain.* Penguin.

FBI. (2008). *Serial murder: Multi-disciplinary perspectives for investigators.* Washington, DC: National Center for the Analysis of Violent Crime.

Ferguson, C. J., Coulson, M., & Barnett, J. (2011). Psychological profiles of school shooters: Positive directions and one big wrong turn. *Journal of Police Crisis Negotiations, 11*(2), 141–158. doi:10.1080/15332586.2011.581523

Fitzgerald, M. (2001). Autistic psychopathy. *Journal of the American Academy of Child and Adolescent Psychiatry, 40*(8), 870. doi:http://dx.doi.org/10.1097/00004583-200108000-00006

Fitzgerald, M. (2010). *Young, violent and dangerous to know.* Hauppauge, NY: Nova Science.

Fitzgerald, M. (2015). *Autism and school shootings—overlap of autism (Asperger's Syndrome) and general psychopathy.* Chapter 1. Retrieved October 15, 2016, from http://cdn.intechopen.com/pdfs-wm/47518.pdf

Follman, M. (2015). *Inside the race to stop the next mass shooter.* Mother Jones. Retrieved December 21, 2016, from http://www.motherjones.com/politics/2015/09/mass-shootings-threat-assessment-shooter-fbi-columbine

Follman, M., Pan, D., & Aronsen, G. (2013, February 27). *A guide to mass shootings in America.* Retrieved from http://www.motherjones.com/special-reports/2012/12/guns-in-america-mass-shootings

Fox, J. A. (2013, January 31). *Responding to Mother Jones.* Retrieved from http://boston.com/community/blogs/crime_punishment/2013/01/responding_to_mother_jones.html

Fox, J. A., & DeLateur, M. J. (2014). Mass shootings in America: Moving beyond Newtown. *Homicide Studies, 18*(1), 125–145. doi:10.1177/1088767913510297

Fox, J. A., & Levin, J. (1994). Firing back: The growing threat of workplace homicide. *The Annals of the American Academy of Political and Social Science, 536*, 16–30. doi:10.1177/0002716294536001002

Fox, J. A., & Levin, J. (2003). Mass murder: An analysis of extreme violence. *Journal of Applied Psychoanalytic Studies, 5*(1), 47–64. doi:10.1023/A:1021051002020

Fox, J. A., & Levin, J. (2015). Mass confusion surrounding mass murder. *The Criminologist, 40*, 8–11.

Gendreau, L. (March 18, 2013). *Sandy hook shooter kept spreadsheet on mass killings: Report.* WVIT. Retrieved February 4, 2016, from http://www.nbcconnecticut.com/news/local/Sandy-Hook-Shooter-Kept-Spreadsheet-on-Mass-Killings-Report-198829761.html

Ghaziuddin, M., Ghaziuddin, N., & Greden, J. (2002). Depression in persons with autism: Implications for research and clinical care. *Journal of Autism and Developmental Disorders, 32*(4), 299–306. doi:10.1023/A:1016330802348

Gillberg, C. (1991). Chapter 4: Clinical and neurobiological aspects of Asperger syndrome in six family studies. *Autism and Asperger Syndrome*, Cambridge: Cambridge University Press, 122–146.

Gillberg, I. C., Helles, A., Billstedt, E., & Gillberg, C. (2016). Boys with Asperger syndrome grow up: Psychiatric and neurodevelopmental disorders 20 years after initial diagnosis. *Journal of Autism and Developmental Disorders, 46*(1), 74–82. doi:10.1007/s10803-015-2544-0

Goodwin, L. (February 19, 2013). *New photos, details emerge of Newtown mass shooter Adam Lanza | The Lookout.* Yahoo! News. Retrieved February 4, 2016, from http://news.yahoo.com/blogs/lookout/photos-details-emerge-newtown-mass-shooter-adam-lanza-124951161.html

Halbfinger, D. M. (December 14, 2012). *A Gunman, Recalled as Intelligent and Shy, Who Left Few Footprints in Life.* The New York Times. Retrieved February 4, 2016, from http://www.nytimes.com/2012/12/15/nyregion/adam-lanza-an-enigma-who-is-now-identified-as-a-mass-killer.html?smid=tw-share&pagewanted=all

Hammond, R. K., & Hoffman, J. M. (2014). Adolescents with high-functioning autism: An investigation of comorbid anxiety and depression. *Journal of Mental Health Research in Intellectual Disabilities, 7*(3), 246–263. doi:10.1080/19315864.2013.843223

Heide, K. M., & Solomon, E. P. (2006). Biology, childhood trauma, and murder: Rethinking justice. *International Journal of Law and Psychiatry, 29*(3), 220–233. doi:10.1016/j.ijlp.2005.10.001

Hempel, A. G., & Richards, T. C. (1999). Offender and offense characteristics of a nonrandom sample of mass murderers. *Journal of the American Academy of Psychiatry and the Law Online, 27*(2), 213–225.

Hinch, R., & Hepburn, C. (1998). Researching serial murder: Methodological and definitional problems. *Electronic Journal of Sociology, 3*(2), 1–11.

Hippler, K., Viding, E., Klicpera, C., & Happé, F. (2010). Brief report: No increase in criminal convictions in Hans Asperger's original cohort. *Journal of Autism and Developmental Disorders, 40*(6), 774–780. doi:10.1007/s10803-009-0917-y

Humphrey, N., & Hebron, J. (2015). Bullying of children and adolescents with autism spectrum conditions: A 'state of the field' review. *International Journal of Inclusive Education, 19*(8), 845–862. doi:10.1080/13603116.2014.981602

Im, D. S. (2016). Template to perpetrate: an update on violence in autism spectrum disorder. *Harvard Review of Psychiatry, 24*(1), 14–35.

Kelly, R. (2010). *Active shooter report: Recommendations and analysis for risk mitigation.* New York, NY: New York City Police Department.

Kerns, C., & Lee, B. (2015). The relationship between adverse childhood experiences and Autism Spectrum Disorder in an epidemiological sample from the United States. *European Psychiatry, 30,* 737. doi:10.1016/S0924-9338(15)30585-X

Kleinfield, N. R., Rivera, R., & Kovaleski, S. F. (March 28, 2013). *Newtown Killer's obsessions, in chilling detail. The New York Times.* Retrieved February 4, 2016, from http://www.nytimes.com/2013/03/29/nyregion/search-warrants-reveal-items-seized-at-adam-lanzas-home.html?_r=0

Kraemer, G. W., Lord, W. D., & Heilbrun, K. (2004). Comparing single and serial homicide offenses. *Behavioral Sciences & the Law, 22*(3), 325–343.

Langman, P. F. (2009). Rampage school shooters: A typology. *Aggression and Violent Behavior, 14,* 79–86. doi:10.1016/j.avb.2008.10.003

Lankford, A. (2015). Are America's public mass shooters unique? A comparative analysis of offenders in the United States and other countries. *International Journal of Comparative and Applied Criminal Justice.* doi:10.1080/01924036.2015.1105144

Lankford, A., & Hakim, N. (2011). From Columbine to Palestine: A comparative analysis of rampage shooters in the USA and volunteer suicide bombers in the Middle East. *Aggression and Violent Behavior, 16,* 98–107. doi:10.1016/j.avb.2010.12.006

Lawrence, R., & Birkland, T. (2004). Guns, Hollywood and school safety: Defining the school-shooting problem across multiple arenas. *Social Science Quarterly, 85,* 1193–1207. doi:10.1111/j.0038-4941.2004.00271.x

Leno, V. C., Charman, T., Pickles, A., Jones, C. R., Baird, G., Happé, F., & Simonoff, E. (2015). Callous–unemotional traits in adolescents with autism spectrum disorder. *The British Journal of Psychiatry, 207*(5), 392–399. doi:10.1192/bjp.bp.114.159863

Levin, J., & Madfis, E. (2009). Mass murder at school and cumulative strain a sequential model. *American Behavioral Scientist, 52*(9), 1227–1245. doi:10.1177/0002764209332543

Lieberman, J. A. (2006). *The shooting game: The making of school shooters.* Santa Ana, CA: Seven Locks Press.

Little, L. (2002). Middle-class mothers' perceptions of peer and sibling victimization among children with Asperger's syndrome and nonverbal learning disorders. *Issues in Comprehensive Pediatric Nursing, 25,* 43–57. doi:10.1080/014608602753504847

Lundström, S., Reichenberg, A., Anckarsäter, H., Lichtenstein, P., & Gillberg, C. (2015). Autism phenotype versus registered diagnosis in Swedish children: Prevalence trends over 10 years in general population samples. *British Medical Journal, 350,* h1961. doi:10.1136/bmj.h1961

Lupica, M. (March 17, 2013). *Lupica: Morbid find suggests murder-obsessed gunman Adam Lanza plotted Newtown, Conn.'s Sandy Hook massacre for years. Daily News.* Retrieved February, 2016, from http://www.nydailynews.com/news/national/lupica-lanza-plotted-massacre-years-article-1.1291408?print

Lysiak, M. (2013). *Newtown: An American Tragedy.* New York: Simon and Schuster.

Maïano, C., Normand, C. L., Salvas, M. C., Moullec, G., & Aimé, A. (2015). Prevalence of school bullying among youth with autism spectrum disorders: A systematic review and meta-analysis. *Autism Research.* doi:10.1002/aur.1568. [Epub ahead of print].

Maras, K., Mulcahy, S., & Crane, L. (2015). Is autism linked to criminality? *Autism, 19*(5), 515–516. doi:10.1177/1362361315583411

Matson, J. L., & Williams, L. W. (2014). Depression and mood disorders among persons with Autism Spectrum Disorders. *Research in Developmental Disabilities, 35*(9), 2003–2007. doi:10.1016/j.ridd.2014.04.020

Metzl, J., & MacLeish, K. (2013). Triggering the debate: Faulty associations between violence and mental illness underlie U.S. gun control efforts. *Risk and Regulation, 25,* 8–10.

Mitchell, K. J., Ybarra, M., & Finkelhor, D. (2007). The relative importance of online victimization in understanding depression, delinquency, and substance use. *Child Maltreatment, 12,* 314–324. doi:10.1177/1077559507305996

Modell, S. J., & Mak, S. (2008). A preliminary assessment of police officers' knowledge and perceptions of persons with disabilities. *Intellectual and Developmental Disabilities, 46,* 183–189. doi:10.1352/2008.46:183-189

Moss, P., Howlin, P., Savage, S., Bolton, P., & Rutter, M. (2015). Self and informant reports of mental health difficulties among adults with autism findings from a long-term follow-up study. *Autism, 19* (7), 832–841. doi:10.1177/1362361315585916

Mouridsen, S. E., Rich, B., Isager, T., & Nedergaard, N. J. (2008). Pervasive developmental disorders and criminal behaviour: A case control study. *International Journal of Offender Therapy and Comparative Criminology, 52*(2), 196–205. doi:10.1177/0306624×07302056

Mukaddes, N. M., & Topcu, Z. (2006). Case report: Homicide by a 10-year-old girl with autistic disorder. *Journal of Autism and Developmental Disorders, 36*(4), 471–474. doi:10.1007/s10803-006-0087-0

Mullen, P. E. (2004). The autogenic (self-generated) massacre. *Behavioral Sciences and the Law, 22*(3), 311–323. doi:10.1002/bsl.564

Murphy, D. (2010). Extreme violence in a man with an autistic spectrum disorder: Assessment and treatment within high-security psychiatric care. *The Journal of Forensic Psychiatry and Psychology, 21*(3), 462–477. doi:10.1080/14789940903426885

Naik, G. (2009). What's on Jim Fallon's mind? A family secret that has been murder to figure out. *The Wall Street Journal.* Retrieved from http://www.wsj.com/articles/SB125745788725531839

Nansel, T. R., Overpeck, M., Haynie, D. L., Ruan, J., & Scheidt, P. C. (2003). Relationships between bullying and violence among US youth. *Archives of Pediatrics and Adolescent Medicine, 157,* 348–353. doi:10.1001/archpedi.157.4.348

Newman, K., & Fox, C. (2009). Repeat tragedy: Rampage shootings in American high school and college settings, 2002–2008). *American Behavioral Scientist, 52,* 1286–1308. doi:10.1177/0002764209332546

Newman, K. S., Fox, C., Roth, W., Mehta, J., & Harding, D. (2004). *Rampage: The social roots of school shootings.* New York, NY: Basic Books.

O'Toole, M. E. (2000). *The school shooter: A threat assessment perspective. Federal Bureau of Investigation.* Retrieved from http://www.fbi.gov/stats-services/publications/school-shooter/

Pilkington, E. (2013). *Sandy Hook report—shooter Adam Lanza was obsessed with mass murder. The Guardian.* November 25, 2013. Retrieved February 4, 2016, from http://www.theguardian.com/world/2013/nov/25/sandy-hook-shooter-adam-lanza-report

Reports: Lanza smashed computer hard drive. USA Today. December 17, 2012. Retrieved February 4, 2016, from http://www.usatoday.com/story/news/nation/2012/12/17/newtown-sandy-hook-adam-lanza-computer-destroyed/1776253/

Rodger, E. (2014a). *FULL VIDEO - Elliot Rodger's retribution video.* Retrieved February 5, 2016, from https://www.youtube.com/watch?v=G-gQ3aAdhIo

Rodger, E. (2014b). *My TWISTED WORLD: The story of Elliot Rodger.* Retrieved February 3, 2016, from http://abclocal.go.com/three/kabc/kabc/My-Twisted-World.pdf

Rugala, E. (2003). *Workplace violence: Issues in response.* Quantico, VA: National Center for the Analysis of Violent Crime, Federal Bureau of Investigation.

Sandy Hook massacre: Adam Lanza acted alone and had an obsession with mass killings. (2013). *The Independent (London).* November 26, 2013. Retrieved February 2016, from http://www.independent.co.uk/news/world/americas/sandy-hook-killer-adam-lanza-acted-alone-and-had-an-obsession-with-mass-killings-such-as-columbine-8963342.html

Schwarz, H., & Ramilo, M. (2014). *Sandy Hook shooter treated at Yale. Yale Daily News.* January 22, 2014. Retrieved February 4, 2016, from http://yaledailynews.com/blog/2014/01/22/sand-hook-shooter-treated-at-yale/

Scragg, P., & Shah, A. (1994). Prevalence of Asperger's syndrome in a secure hospital. *The British Journal of Psychiatry, 165*(5), 679–682. doi:10.1192/bjp.165.5.679

Sedensky, S. J. (2013). *Sandy hook final report. Office of the State's attorney, judicial district of Danbury.* Stephen J. Sedensky III, State's Attorney November 25, 2013. Retrieved February 2016, http://www.ct.gov/csao/lib/csao/Sandy_Hook_Final_Report.pdf

Silva, J. A., Leong, G. B., & Ferrari, M. M. (2004). A neuropsychiatric developmental model of serial homicidal behavior. *Behavioral Sciences and The Law, 22*(6), 787–799. doi:10.1002/bsl.620

Skrapec, C. A. (2001). Defining serial murder: A call for a return to the original Lustmörd. *Journal of Police and Criminal Psychology, 16*(2), 10–24. doi:10.1007/BF02805177

Sobsey, D., Wells, D., Lucardie, R., & Mansell, S. (Eds.) (1995). *Violence and disability: An annotated bibliography.* Baltimore, MD: Brookes.

Solomon, A. (2014). *"The Reckoning". The New Yorker (New Yorker).* March 17, 2014. Retrieved February 4, 2016 from http://www.newyorker.com/magazine/2014/03/17/the-reckoning

Taylor, M. J., Charman, T., & Ronald, A. (2015). Where are the strongest associations between autistic traits and traits of ADHD? Evidence from a community-based twin study. *European Child and Adolescent Psychiatry, 24*(9), 1129–1138. doi:10.1007/s00787-014-0666-0.

The Secret Life Of Elliot Rodger Interview. (2014). Retrieved February 5, 2016, from https://www.youtube.com/watch?vDpnT0CMwBrWs

Vossekuil, B., Fein, R., Reddy, M., Borum, R., & Modzeleski, W. (2002). *The final report and findings of the safe school initiative: Implications for the prevention of school attacks in the United States.* Washington, DC: United States Secret Service and United States Department of Education.

Wainscot, J. J., Naylor, P., Sutcliffe, P., Tantam, D., & Williams, J. V. (2008). Relationships with peers and use of the school environment of mainstream secondary school pupils with Asperger Syndrome (High- Functioning Autism): A case-control study. *International Journal of Psychology and Psychological Therapy, 8*, 25–38.

Winter, T., Rappleye, H., Alba, M., & Dahlgren, K. (2013). *Police release full Newtown massacre report, with photos and video—Investigations.* NBC News. December 27, 2013. Retrieved February 4, 2016, from http://investigations.nbcnews.com/_news/2013/12/27/21736461-police-release-full-newtown-massacre-report-with-photos-and-video?lite

Woodbury-Smith, M. R., Clare, I. C. H., Holland, A. J., & Kearns, A. (2006). High functioning autistic spectrum disorders, offending and other law-breaking: Findings from a community sample. *The Journal of Forensic Psychiatry and Psychology, 17*(1), 108–120. doi:10.1080/14789940600589464

Yaksic, E. (2015). Addressing the challenges and limitations of utilizing data to study serial homicide. *Crime Psychology Review, 1*(1), 108–134.

Ybarra, M. L., & Mitchell, K. J. (2004). Online aggressor/targets, aggressors, and targets: A comparison of associated youth characteristics. *Journal of Child Psychology and Psychiatry, 45*, 1308–1316. doi:10.1111/j.1469-7610.2004.00328.x

# Senseless Violence Against Central American Unaccompanied Minors: Historical Background and Call for Help

Cheryl B. Sawyer and Judith Márquez

**ABSTRACT**

The southwestern U.S. border has recently seen a significant increase in the number of unaccompanied children from Honduras, Guatemala, and El Salvador illegally crossing the Mexican border into the United States. Many of these children leave home to flee violence, starvation, impoverished living conditions, or other life-threatening situations. The treatment of acute stress, anxiety, and depression associated with traumatic events is crucial in helping these children address these negative psychological events they have experienced so that they can move forward with their lives. Untreated, traumatic events experienced by this population can develop into Post Traumatic Stress Disorder, a potentially life-changing and physically threatening psychological and medical issue. The United States needs to effectively address the serious matter of responding to mental health issues facing refugees from war-torn or impoverished nations so as to help them to successfully adjust to American systems. There is a need for researchers in the mental health field to focus efforts in designing, implementing, and evaluating methodologies that can help these children develop healthy strategies for living with a very difficult and complex past.

The united nations estimates the displaced refugee worldwide population was approximately 59.5 million people in 2014 (United Nations Refugee Agency, 2014). While much global attention has been focused on providing support for Europe's burgeoning refugee crisis, the Central American refugee crisis in the United States has resulted in significant political controversy. This wave of refugees is being treated as so many other refugees have been treated when they make their way to the United States. They face rejection, deportation, and discrimination. Despite the animosity that awaits them, more than 60,000 unaccompanied, undocumented children suffered incredible hardships and risk to cross the Mexican border into Texas during 2014. To better understand the crisis, Americans need to have a grasp of who is crossing our Southwestern borders and the reasons why these children are placing their lives in jeopardy to flee their homeland. The purpose of this article is to give the reader an overview of the history behind the unaccompanied minor immigration movement and to help the reader understand the stresses, struggles, and obstacles as well as the strengths of these individuals.

## Historical perspective of Central American political dysfunction

Although the issues associated with Central American political unrest are vastly complex, it is helpful to have a basic understanding of the underlying political and socioeconomic history of the area in order to better grasp the current situation. Each of the three countries in Central America's northern triangle, Honduras, El Salvador, and Guatemala, have a history of extreme violence and civil unrest.

### Honduras

A military coup in Honduras shut down opposition with excessive force in 2009. At that time, the government suspended freedom of assembly and freedom of the press and authorized excessive force on peaceful demonstrations. The governmental police continued to be highly corrupt. Police killed at least 149 civilians in 2011–2012, yet few were subject to investigation. The U.S. State Department continues to monitor the Honduran government, especially the Honduran National Police. The United States has held back portions of financial aid until the Honduran government fulfills several human rights requirements. Crime appears to go unchecked and unprosecuted, particularly against journalists, LGBTI, and peasants. Prisons are overcrowded, filled at approximately 33% past capacity (PBS, 2011). International criminal gangs such as the 18th Street gang and the MS-13 gang are well armed and actively involved in murder, kidnapping, extortion, execution-for-hire, carjacking, narco-trafficking, armed robbery, and home invasions (Overseas Security Advisory Council, 2016a). Street crime is rampant and rarely prosecuted (Overseas Security Advisory Council, 2016b).

### El Salvador

Throughout the 1980s and into the early 1990s, a vicious civil war occurred between the Farabundo Martí National Liberation Front (FMLN), one of the Salvadorian political parties, and the government of El Salvador. The United States supported the Salvadorian government with the hope that a moderate government could form a stable economic and political foundation. The FMLN, supported by Cuban, Soviet, and Nicaraguan governments, utilized guerilla warfare and terrorist tactics to intimidate citizens into joining their efforts. Mayors, priests, informants, and others perceived as traitors to the cause were executed; death squads executed entire families and decapitation by machete was common (Allison, 2012; Torres, 2014). The war spilled over into neighboring Nicaragua and Honduras, countries that were also leaning toward communistic views (Torres, 2014). Peace talks were held in 1992; the FMLN became the leading political party and gained control of the government. The ability of the FMLN to curb the violently charged atmosphere of the 1980s civil war era is described as marginal, at best (Farah, 2016).

As a result of the violent political climate, massive numbers of people fled the country: army deserters, guerilla fighters, and many families all fled El Salvador during the civil war. Many came to the United States and settled in the Los Angeles area in the Latino neighborhoods. The names of the gangs originated from the street names that defined their territories. The best known of the gangs, the Mara-Salvatrucha-13 (MS-13) organization, was formed by Salvadorian refugees as protection against rival Mexican, African American, and Chinese gangs (Garsd, 2015; Torres, 2014).

## Guatemala

Guatemala still suffers massive repercussions as a continued legacy of a 36-year civil war. The U.S. Central Intelligence Agency supported a coup in 1954 in which poor farmers lost both their lands and voting rights. This action eventually led to grass-roots guerilla warfare against governmental military forces that began in 1960 and continued until 1996. During the next 36 years, the country alternated between civilian and military rule, multiple coups coupled with a dissolved constitution, Congress, and Supreme Court. More than 200,000 people were killed. The abductions, murders, mutilations, public dumping of bodies, rape, extortion, and intimidation that were prevalent during the civil war have continued; organized crime and gangs operate openly and continue to paralyze the country. Although many gang members have been imprisoned, the prisons appear to serve as central hubs from which continued crime is orchestrated and directed. Women and girls are particularly targeted; hundreds have been abducted and taken to prisons where they were raped by prisoners under the supervision of highly corrupt prison officials (PBS, 2011).

## The violence continues

Reports of street fighting within these small Central American countries are intensifying. In 2013, the murder rate in Honduras was cited as the highest in the world (PBS, 2011). The death rate for El Salvador is currently estimated to be approximately 105:100,000 citizens, the highest in the world (Farah, 2016). El Salvador's population is less than that of New York City, yet it still averages approximately 30 murders each day (Garsd, 2015). More than 100 battles have already been fought in 2016 between police and street gangs; police are reported to be abandoning their posts due to insufficient support and equipment (Ditta, 2016). The Salvadorian minister of security has given police the authority to shoot perceived gang members on sight (Ditta, 2016). The MS-13 are now crucial players in the transportation of cocaine out of South America into Mexico and the United States. The MS-13 are categorized by the Federal Bureau of Investigation as a medium to high threat within the United States. They tend to recruit middle and high school children with activities that include rape, prostitution, drug distribution, kidnapping, sex trafficking; they are known to be active in at least 42 states (FBI, 2008). A rival gang, the 18th Street Gang, is currently active in all three northern triangle countries: Guatemala, Honduras, and El Salvador (Seelke, 2016).

The violence has infiltrated all aspects of society but primarily focuses within poor neighborhoods. Children as young as 7 or 8 are recruited by gangs; girls are kidnapped, used as objects, and discarded. For instance, one 15-year old girl was shot at close range for selling tortillas in another gang's territory. Another 15-year old girl was attacked from behind and shot twice in the head while walking on the street because her boyfriend avoided joining the gang. Another girl is afraid to leave the house; after her best friend simply disappeared and her family moved away, hiding from the gangs (Garsd, 2015) . Another girl was threatened by her own father, a gang member who is now in prison. He has threatened to rape and kill her when he gets out of prison unless her mother gives him $50,000 (Garsd, 2015). A 22-year old man who left home to deliver his family's rent money was found dead in a ditch, hands and feet cut off (Nazario, 2015).

Children roam hungry, and poverty is rampant in many neighborhoods. Mothers, unwilling to watch their children starve, abandon their children to come to the United States seeking employment so that they can send money to their home country so that their children can eat.

## Undocumented, unaccompanied children come to the United States

Over the past few years, the southwestern border of the United States, primarily in Texas, has seen a significant increase in the number of undocumented, accompanied children from Honduras, Guatemala, and El Salvador illegally crossing the Mexican border into the United States (U.S. Customs and Border Protection, 2015). Authorities estimate that between 65,000 and 90,000 undocumented, unaccompanied children attempted this journey between 2012–2014 (U.S. Customs and Border Protection, 2015). Many of these children leave their homes to flee violence, starvation, impoverished living conditions, or other life threatening situations. In the minds of these children, the dangerous conditions of their native land are more pressing than the perils involved in the actual journey and subsequent immigration issues (Nazario, 2014). The journey itself is complex and highly dangerous, often including jumping onto and riding the tops of freight trains. The children also face potential kidnapping, rape, mutilation, incarceration, beating, and other traumatic events. Once the child reaches the Rio Grande River, the division between Texas and Mexico, the potential for abuse, capture, enslavement, or even death continues, as the child must negotiate the illegal border crossing into Texas. Smugglers (called coyotes), Border Patrol, cartels/gangs, and American vigilantes all seek this vulnerable population in hopes of apprehending them (Nazario, 2014).

Many of these children are apprehended by U.S. authorities and placed in holding facilities pending disposition by a judge. These children may be detained for a considerable amount of time while the judicial system determines whether they will be deported or permitted to stay in the United States; placement with an appropriate family in the United States can take additional time. Even if the children are reunited with families in the United States, problems associated with abandonment and trauma coupled with adjustment to life in the United States can pose obstacles for the child's potential success in the United States (Pierce, 2015).

## U.S. political response

In 2015, U.S. representatives met with officials from El Salvador, Guatemala, Honduras, and Mexico to formulate a plan to halt the massive influx of refugees and ultimately provided Mexico with substantial funding designated for support in halting the refugees at its southern border. This action has provided the funding for an additional level of violence: Mexican state and federal police, many open to bribery and corruption, now have a monetary incentive for stopping the refugees and use whatever resources available to stop the children from northward migration. Mexico has instituted physical deterrents to prevent northern migration, such as low hanging structures designed to knock refugees from the roofs of trains, and concrete pillars on the sides of tracks to prevent children from running along the sides of the moving trains. In the last six months of 2015, U.S. funds resulted in Mexico's deployment of 300–600 immigration agents who conducted 20,000 raids, and apprehended 92,889 Central American refugees; some refugees tell of police who killed, raped, beat, or robbed refugees seeking asylum (Nazario, 2015). Nazario (2015) has stressed that Mexican officials can account for more than 72,000 refugees that were rescued from kidnappers over the past few years. These survivors describe being forced into prostitution or farming in the marijuana fields; some survivors told stories about individuals who were murdered and their organs harvested. Even these obstacles do not seem to effectively deter the children from migrating northward into the United States. Mexico only granted asylum to 18 children in 2014 (Nazario, 2015). In the first seven months of 2015, U.S. officials apprehended 70,448 Central American refugees.

## Psychological and Ecological Implications and Recommendations

There is a need to better understand the stresses, struggles, and obstacles as well as the strengths of these individuals in order to develop effective practices for helping these individuals obtain success in the United States. Many refugee children who enter this country have severe complex trauma, limited ability to speak English, sporadic opportunities for education, and few resources for coping with life in a new country. Treating the acute stress, anxiety, and depression associated with traumatic events is crucial for helping these children address these negative psychological events so that they can move forward with their lives (Barber, Kohn, Kassam-Adams, & Gold, 2014). Untreated, traumatic events experienced by this population can develop into Post Traumatic Stress Disorder (PTSD), a potentially life-changing and physically threatening psychological and medical issue (Barber et al., 2014; D'Andrea, Ford, Stolbach, Spinazzola, & van der Kolk, 2012). These children are at high risk for psychological and behavioral problems. Depression, hypervigilance, sleeping disorders, psychotic episodes, and unpredictable moods only touch the surface of the challenges these children face.

Culturally competent mental health services in the child's native language are sparse (Pierce, 2015). Mental health counselors and therapists are currently seeking to remediate this issue by exploring and documenting various treatment methods. In October 2014, in an attempt to bring together those practitioners and researchers who have been working with the aforementioned population, the National Latino Psychology Association (NLPA) organized an international conference entitled Dreamers, Immigration, and Social Justice: Advancing a Global Latina/o Psychology Agenda. Presentations at this conference (Arciniega, 2014; Gómez-Marmolejo, Karraa, Estrada, & Rodríguez, 2014; López, 2014; Paz & Barcenas, 2014; Ramos & Hawley-McWhirter, 2014) stressed that these children need to be able to tell the story of their trauma in a nonthreatening manner as part of the therapeutic process. Future NLPA Conferences, such as the 2016 conference—Advocating for Social Justice, Liberation, and Equality for Familias—have the potential for further expanding the current body of research surrounding techniques and strategies for addressing mental health issues. All mental health associations might seriously consider following this organization's lead and encourage research presentations related to this population as a priority for future national conferences and publications. Preliminary results of research conducted by the University of Houston-Clear Lake Counselor Training program indicate that narrative storytelling using the client's native language in a safe, nonthreatening setting has the potential for reducing some of the fears and confusion related to the trauma involved in the type of immigration experiences unaccompanied minors have faced.

## Conclusion

The United States needs to more effectively address the serious issue of responding to mental health problems experienced by refugees from war-torn or impoverished nations to help them successfully adjust to American systems. The United States cannot simply avoid the crisis by deporting the refugees. While many politicians eschew these refugees and work toward deporting them as quickly as possible, data show that nearly 98% of these children ultimately remain in the country (Tate, 2014).

Researchers in the mental health field need to focus efforts on designing, implementing, and evaluating methodologies that can help these refugees develop healthy strategies for living with very difficult and complex experiences. Although a review of the literature offers some suggestions for providing mental health support for refugees from Eastern Europe, the Middle East, and the African continent, a minimal amount has been published in the field related to providing mental health support for Central American refugees. Mental health counselors and therapists are currently seeking to remediate this issue by exploring and documenting various treatment methods. Changes in governmental policy, mental health support, and education that can effectively provide viable solutions for this crisis need to be developed and implemented.

## References

Allison, M. (2012). *El Salvador's brutal civil war: What we still don't know*. Retrieved from http://www. aljazeera.com/indepth/opinion/2012/02/2012228123122975116.html

Arciniega, M. (2014). *A holistic approach to counseling undocumented students*. Paper presented at National Latino Psychologist Association Biennial Conference: Albuquerque, N.M. Retrieved from http://www.nlpa.ws/assets/nlpa2014%20program%20final.pdf

Barber, B. A., Kohl, K. L., Kassam-Adams, N., & Gold, J. I. (2014). Acute stress, depression, and anxiety symptoms among English and Spanish-speaking children with recent trauma exposure. *Journal of Clinical Psychology in Medical Settings, 21*(1), 66–71.

D'Andrea, W., Ford, J., Stolbach, B., Spinazzola, J., & van der Kolk, B. A. (2012). Understanding interpersonal trauma in children: Why we need a developmentally appropriate trauma diagnosis. *American Journal of Orthopsychiatry, 82*(2), 187–200.

Ditta, E. (2016). *3 to 4 gun battles a day: El Salvador police chief*. Retrieved from http://www.insight crime.org/news-briefs/three-to-four-gun-battles-a-day-el-salvador-police

Farah, D. (2016). *Central America's gangs are all grown up and more dangerous than ever*. Retrieved from http://foreignpolicy.com/2016/01/19/central-americas-gangs-are-all-grown-up

Federal Bureau of Investigation (FBI). (2008). *The MS-13 threat: A national assessment*. Retrieved from https://www.fbi.gov/news/stories/2008/january/ms13_011408

Garsd, J. (2015). *How El Salvador fell into a web of gang violence*. Retrieved from http://www.npr.org/sections/goatsandsoda/2015/10/05/445382231/how-el-salvador-fell-into-a-web-of-gang-violence

Gómez-Marmolejo, P. M., Karraa, S., Estrada, M., & Rodríguez, C. (2014). *Resilience and depression in refugee children separated by the deportation of their parents*. Poster session presented at National Latino Psychologist Association Biennial Conference: Albuquerque, NM. Retrieved from http://www.nlpa.ws/assets/nlpa2014%20program%20final.pdf

López, G. (2014). *Posttraumatic growth in unaccompanied undocumented minors from Central American countries*. Paper presented at National Latino Psychologist Association Biennial Conference: Albuquerque, N.M. Retrieved from http://www.nlpa.ws/assets/nlpa2014%20program%20final.pdf

Nazario, S. (2014). Enrique's journey. New York: Random House.

Nazario, S. (2015). *Refugees at our door*. *New York Times*. Retrieved from http://www.nytimes.com/2015/10/11/opinion/sunday/the-refugees-at-our-door.html?_r=0

Overseas Security Advisory Council. (2016a). *Guatemala 2015 crime and safety report*. United States Department of State: Bureau of Diplomatic Security. Retrieved from http://www.osac.gov/ContentReportDetails.aspx?cid=17494

Overseas Security Advisory Council. (2016b). *Honduras 2015 crime and safety report*. *United States Department of State: Bureau of Diplomatic Security*. Retrieved from http://www.osac.gov/ContentReportDetails.aspx?cid=17494

Paz, M., & Barcenas, G. (2014). *Dynamic dimensions of working with Latino children and their families in elementary schools*. Symposium presented at National Latino Psychologist Association Biennial Conference: Albuquerque, N.M. Retrieved from http://www.nlpa.ws/assets/nlpa2014%20program%20final.pdf

Pierce, S. (2015). Unaccompanied child refugees in U.S. communities, immigration court, and schools. *Migration Policy Institute*. Retrieved from http://www.migrationpolicy.org/research/unaccompanied-child-migrants-us-communities-immigration-court-and-schools

Public Broadcasting Systems (PBS). (2011). *Timeline: Guatemala's brutal civil war*. Retrieved from http://www.pbs.org/newshour/updates/latin_america-jan-june11-timeline_03-07/

Ramos, K., & Hawley-McWhirter. (2014). *First-generation Latino immigrant students: Exploring the relationship between migration experience and education outcomes*. Poster session presented at National Latino Psychologist Association Biennial Conference: Albuquerque, N.M. Retrieved from http://www.nlpa.ws/assets/nlpa2014%20program%20final.pdf

Seelke, C. (2016). *CRS report for Congress: Gangs in Central America*. Retrieved from https://www.fas.org/sgp/crs/row/RL34112.pdf

Tate, J. (2014). *Mexico stopped flow of undocumented minors prior to US elections*. *Breitbart News Network*. Retrieved from http://www.breitbart.com/texas/2014/12/08/mexico-stopped-flow-of-undocumented-minors-prior-to-us-elections/

Torres, A. (2014). *History of the Mara Salvatrucha gang: Anti-authoritarian attitudes and outlandish gang tattoos characterize members*. Retrieved from http://www.local10.com/news/history-of-the-mara-salvatrucha-gang

United Nations Refugee Agency. (2014). *UNHCR global trends: Forced displacement in 2014*. Retrieved from http://unhcr.org/556725e69.html#_ga=1.252785929.1851762221.1456428723

U.S. Customs & Border Protection. (2015). Southwest border unaccompanied alien children apprehensions Fiscal Year 2016. Retrieved from https://www.cbp.gov/newsroom/stats/southwest-border-unaccompanied-children/fy-2016

# Violent Video Games Exposed: A Blow by Blow Account of Senseless Violence in Games

Andrew Krantz, Vipul Shukla, Michele Knox, and Karyssa Schrouder

**ABSTRACT**

Violent video game (VVG) use has repeatedly been found to be associated with hostile expectations about others, desensitization to violence, decreased empathy and prosocial behavior, and aggressive thoughts and behaviors. Although these research findings have been widely publicized, VVGs remain the most extensively played games and represent a multi-billion dollar industry. Although VVGs are typically rated "mature," indicating they are not suitable for youths, they are often purchased for youths. This may be in part because there is currently no system available to consumers that thoroughly describes the content of video games, and much of the public is unaware of the types of violence that characterize game play. The purpose of this paper is to describe the violent content of some of the top VVGs, based on sales. For the purposes of this issue, acts of senseless, unprovoked violence will be described in detail.

Video game play is an avid hobby for many people in the United States. In fact, today, approximately 40% of young adults play violent video games (VVGs) every week or more often (Padilla-Walker, Nelson, Carroll, & Jensen, 2010). Furthermore, most American youths aged between 8 and 18 years play video games at least occasionally (Gentile, 2009). Media use by children and youths typically is not supervised, and less than half of the children said that their parents or caregivers have rules or limits about their game play (Rideout, Foehr, & Roberts, 2010). In studies conducted since the popularity of video games has exploded, children and adolescents frequently report that their parents do not monitor or restrict their use of technology (Strasburger & Donnerstein, 1999). Even if parents are somewhat aware of their children's activity, they underreport hours of use and anything problematic with what they are using (Strasburger & Donnerstein, 1999). In fact, 90% of teenagers say their parents never check the rating before allowing them to buy or rent a video game (Walsh, 2000). Even more, teenagers often play video games that give players access to additional material through website codes, bonus material that often is not included in the rating of the game (Haninger & Thompson, 2004; Brekke, 2006). Compared to television and movies, video games are the second least-monitored media activity after television (Roberts, 1999).

The potential effects of video games on players have been studied extensively. In a meta-analytic review, for example, VVG use was positively associated with aggressive behavior, aggressive cognitions, and aggressive affect (Anderson et al., 2010; Bushman & Huesmann, 2006). VVG use has been demonstrated to relate to increases in aggressive behavior in youths, and increased VVG play is associated with higher levels of aggression over time (Anderson et al., 2010). Also, results of meta-analyses demonstrate associations between VVG play and desensitization to violence, decreased empathy and decreased prosocial behavior (Anderson et al., 2010).

Since video game play has become so prevalent, methods to educate the public about the appropriateness and content of games have been explored. For example, the Entertainment Software Rating Board (ESRB) is a self-regulatory body founded by the Interactive Digital Software Association (IDSA). The leading video game manufacturers developed the ESRB in response to publicly stated concerns over the content of video games. The ESRB informs the public whether or not games include content such as sex, violence, profanity, and substance use. The ESRB gives age recommendations for the games (ESRB, 2016). Today, most of the top-selling video games carry a rating of "Mature" (M) or "Teen" (T). According to the ESRB, in T-rated games, "content is generally suitable for ages 13 and up. May contain violence, suggestive themes, crude humor, minimal blood, simulated gambling and/or infrequent use of strong language" (ESRB, 2016). In M-rated games, "content is generally suitable for ages 17 and up.... May contain intense violence, blood and gore, sexual content and/or strong language" (ESRB, 2016).

Even though these content ratings are available, many buyers do not use them. For example, as demonstrated in the Walsh (2000) study, 90% of teens say their parents do not check video game ratings before purchase. Parents, who may want to limit their child's exposure to violent video games, often are thwarted by the inconsistency between rating systems for various other media products (Gentile & Walsh, 2002). Because of this inconsistency and lack of knowledge, parents often fail to use ratings consistently or at all (Gentile & Walsh, 2002). In their 2002 study, Gentile and Walsh found that only "25% of parents always use industry ratings to select appropriate games" (p. 170). However, even if parents were to use the age-based labels, "the disparity between the existing age ratings and the age-appropriate standards of most parents, which do not achieve consensus themselves, suggests that the age based ratings are founded on a false consensus of what is age appropriate" (Gentile, Maier, Hasson, & Bonetti, 2011, p. 42). This suggests that the game content may still be inappropriate from some parents' perspectives, further adding to the confusion. Another group (Bijvank, Konjin, Bushman, & Roelofsma, 2009) found that, "age-based labels and violence content labels only made video games more attractive, like forbidden fruits. The more restrictive, the more attractive...." (p. 874). In contrast, knowing details about the content may allow children to make better, more informed decisions, because "content-based ratings are more likely to decrease [the child's interest] (the "tainted fruit" effect)" (Gentile et al., 2011; p. 42).

The one point of agreement between parents and industry ratings is with ratings for products labeled as unsuitable for children (R-rated movies, mature audience (MA) shows, etc.); beyond this, industry ratings are too lenient compared to how parents rate the same product (Walsh & Gentile, 2001). Parents want a more specific, content-based ratings system, not simple categories (Gentile et al., 2011). Thus, although the current rating systems provide broad categories of potentially problematic or objectionable content, they give the buyer insufficient detail to make informed decisions about the games.

One study compared three previous survey-driven studies to clarify what parents want from a potential revamp of rating systems (Gentile et al., 2011). The findings demonstrated that parents are aware that the existing ratings do not provide all of the information they want, are not accurate, and are not often used. Content descriptors most asked for were sexual content, violence, language, and mature content on a broad scale, with more specific situations labeled underneath. Because there is no consensus on age-based ratings, content-based ratings may work better for most parents, allowing them to judge what is and is not appropriate for their child. Furthermore, with content-based rating systems, there would be less chance for "ratings creep" (shift over time for more mature content to get to lower age-based ratings), because they would be designed to precisely report the presence or absence of specific content.

In a 2011 study, researchers found that "parents who understood video games rating system were more likely to prohibit their use due to rating" (Colón-de Marti, Rodriguez-Figueroa, Gutierrez, & Gonzalez, 2011, p. 23). Haninger and Thompson (2004) advocate for the same parental insight, "Parents need not necessarily play the games; they can easily observe and be part of their child's experience" (p. 865). In a study focused more on ratings for television, it was found that for younger children, "involvement may encourage children to internalize their parents' viewing standards" (Cantor, 1998, p. 64Gentile and Walsh (2002) add support to this practice of active mediation by finding that it positively influences how a child internalizes information from the media, and other experts have concurred that encouraging parents' involvement in media viewing may be the best way to influence a child's critical viewing skills (Abelman, 1990).

Some research has been conducted to examine in more detail the content of video games (e.g., Smith, 2006). In one study on T-rated games, for example, 98% of the games studied were reported to involve intentional violence, 90% encouraged or required the player to injure characters, 69% encouraged or required the player to kill, 27% depicted sexual themes, 27% had profanity, and 15% depicted intoxicating substances. Games were significantly more likely to depict females partially nude or engaged in sexual behaviors than males (Haninger & Thompson, 2004). Furthermore, M-rated video games were significantly more likely to contain blood, profanity, and substance use, to show more severe injuries, and to have a higher rate of deaths than video games rated T (Thompson, Tepichin, & Haninger, 2006). In one study, content was found to relate to intention; when the blood manipulation was on (that is, the player is able to control whether or not blood is visible on themselves and/or other characters while playing the game), players reported increased intent to be physically aggressive (Weber, Ritterfeld, & Mathiak, 2006). One genre of VVG that has been described is the "atmosphere game" that depicts and promotes a generally violent world or atmosphere. Atmosphere games contain senseless violence that is necessary to achieve the goal of the game. For example, one game is described as "letting people live out their socio-pathic fantasies" and awarding points according to how much mayhem the player causes (Reeves, 2009, p. 522–523). Although a minimal amount has been published on sexual acts in video games, gender role stereotyping and an emphasis on sexuality of women depicted in video games has been described in detail (e.g., Downs & Smith, 2010; Beasley & Collins Standley, 2002).

Some research has indicated that the content of games may be associated with outcomes. For example, profanity used by game characters has been shown to increase gamers' hostile expectations of others, potentially contributing to an increased likelihood of aggressive behavior (Ivory & Kaestle, 2013). Characteristics of games that promote emotional disengagement in players have been studied and hypothesized to relate to associations between VVG play and aggressive behavior. For example, findings from a recent study suggested that moral disengagement factors are often included in first-person shooter games, and VVGs often include justifications for violence, a distorted portrayal of the consequences of violent acts, and dehumanization of victims (Hartmann, Krakowiak, & Tsay-Vogel, 2014). If the content of VVGs predicts outcomes for players, then game content and characteristics are clearly topics worthy of further study and disclosure.

The published content studies have provided valuable information to researchers and consumers about the components of games. However, video game content changes rapidly as developers produce new products, and consumer demand for newer and better games increases. Consumers, especially avid players, become accustomed to the content of games, and appetites increase for bold, unforeseen content, improved graphics, and innovative themes. Until a reliable, publicly accessible system for detailed descriptions of complete game content exists, it will be important to regularly research and publicize information about content. Such research would provide descriptions of the various violent acts in games, many of which are unusual and not readily conceived by the public. Knowledge of this violent content is important for players and buyers of games who may believe the types virtual violence experienced in VVGs to be something more common (e.g., hitting, pushing) and less harmful than is in fact the case (e.g., torture, mass shootings). That is, although buyers and players may know that violence is in the games, they may not be aware of, or prepared for, the brutality and inhumane acts therein. Secondly, engaging in these acts during the VVG play allows players to form new conceptions for violent acts. For example, one of the ways that VVGs are thought to promote violent behavior is through the development and increased accessibility of cognitive scripts for violent behavior (Anderson, 2003). That is, VVG players are able to conceive of, imagine, or picture violent acts that they see in games. Playing the game "primes" those scripts, making them more cognitively available to the player both during and after game play. If games now include content depicting acts such as physical beatings, torture, and mass shootings, then players may be more likely to develop scripts for such behaviors, whereas if they had not played the game, they would not have such scripts. For example, children who had never conceived of torture may become newly aware of this concept and form a torture "script" after playing the video game with this content. Adults who had never conceived of committing mass shootings may begin to consider such. In addition, the games promote hostile knowledge and belief systems that contribute to players' beliefs that the world is a dangerous place, that conflict should be handled with aggression, and that aggression is an effective way to meet one's goals (Bushman & Anderson, 2002).

In summary, VVG play is highly prevalent and research indicates a host of negative outcomes associated with VVG exposure. Especially concerning are the potential impacts of VVG play on youths. Nonetheless, VVG play continues to grow. The content of games appears to relate to outcomes experienced by players. Despite this, publicly accessible information about game content is limited, and parents, caregivers, and others who buy VVGs for youths are often making uninformed choices. The present study aims to provide detailed qualitative reports on the violent content in video games. Specifically, the study provides a detailed description of the senseless acts of violence in top-selling violent video games of the previous fiscal year. The study provides a

**Table 1.** Thematic content and descriptions of ESRB game-ratings (ESRB, 2016).

| ESRB Content | Description |
| --- | --- |
| Blood and Gore | Depictions of blood or the mutilation of body parts |
| Drug Reference | Reference to and/or images of illegal drugs |
| Intense Violence | Graphic and realistic-looking depictions of physical conflict. May involve extreme and/or realistic blood, gore, weapons, and depictions of human injury and death |
| Language | Mild to moderate use of profanity |
| Mature Humor | Depictions or dialogue involving "adult" humor, including sexual references |
| Nudity | Graphic or prolonged depictions of nudity |
| Sexual Content | Nonexplicit depictions of sexual behavior, possibly including partial nudity |
| Sexual Violence | Depictions of rape or other violent sexual acts |
| Strong Language | Explicit and/or frequent use of profanity |
| Violence | Scenes involving aggressive conflict. May contain bloodless dismemberment |

novel description of video game violence, because it describes acts in later parts of games that have not been described previously. Because previous studies have quantified acts of violence, this study endeavored to provide a more qualitative description, a "play-by-play" of acts of senseless violence for people who have not played the games. This study can serve as insight into the kinds of VVG content that are increasingly available to game players, so that the public can be more aware of the types, levels, and contexts of senseless violence that players can access in video games.

## Methods

Six top selling home-console video games were selected from games released from 2013. Video games selected were identified as containing violence, blood, and language in content descriptions and ESRB ratings (Table 1). All games selected were contained within a recently published list of the top twenty games based on sales in the fiscal year 2015 (Ranj, 2016). Researchers conducted two trials for each selected game; trials consisted of two researchers alternating between playing the video game for two-hour intervals and recording in detail instances of unprovoked acts of violence. While one researcher would play the selected game, the other would observe and record detailed descriptions of gameplay from the trial. These descriptions focused on violent scenes from the games, and included narrative context and the style of gameplay. Observations regarding violent content were compared to the ratings and content descriptors used by the ESRB (Table 1), and those ratings and content descriptors assigned to the games by the ESRB (Table 2). Discretion was used in cases where the acts of violence did not clearly fall under the operational definition of unprovoked.

For the purposes of this study the researchers extended the definition of senseless violence to include unprovoked acts, as the word "senseless" may not fully imply the context of certain actions. As defined by the Oxford English Dictionary, "unprovoked" refers to "an attack or a display of aggression or emotion not caused by anything done or said" (Oxford Dictionaries, 2016). For the sake of our study, unprovoked acts of violence were defined as acts that were not predicated on self-defense (e.g., retaliation as a means avoiding further personal harm), political motivation (e.g., acts of warfare for military or political gain), or overt monetary compensation (e.g., "hitman" scenarios). Following with this definition, unprovoked acts of violence were considered to be those with no clear motivation, or where the proportionality of violence grossly outweighed any political or monetary motivation.

**Table 2.** ESRB ratings and content descriptors for games played (ESRB, 2016).

| Game | ESRB Rating | Content Descriptors |
|---|---|---|
| 1 | M (Mature) | Blood and Gore, Intense Violence, Mature Humor, Nudity, Strong Language, Strong Sexual Content, Use of Drugs and Alcohol |
| 2 | T (Teen) | Blood, Mild Language, Violence |
| 3 | M (Mature) | Blood and Gore, Drug Reference, Intense Violence, Strong Language |
| 4 | T (Teen) | Animated Blood, Violence |
| 5 | M (Mature) | Blood and Gore, Intense Violence, Sexual Themes, Strong Language |
| 6 | M (Mature) | Blood and Gore, Intense Violence, Strong Language |

## Results

The first playing session involved a home-console game directed in the third person—otherwise referred to as a "third-person shooter" (TPS)—that offered the player a variety of violent courses of action to be used at the player's discretion. The game included elements of massive multi-player online role-playing games (MMORPG), first-person shooter (FPS), and driving games, although the central themes revolved around violent and explicitly criminal activity. The nature of the gameplay is such that a player can interact with the storyline and content based on their personal preferences, rather than following a strict narrative progression. Given the options of camera angles, the researchers decided to play in the TPS mode rather than from a first-person point of view. During the course of gameplay, researchers were given a range of narrative opportunities that ranged from leisurely activities such as skydiving to "jobs" and "missions" that included, but were not limited to, assassinations, unprovoked killing sprees, arms trafficking, and interrogation by means of torture. In order to fully serve the intent of this study, researchers opted for violent gameplay as it presented itself. In turn, researchers were frequently able to engage in unprovoked physical beatings of other subjects in the game, as well as shootings, vehicular homicide, and armed robbery.

While this game presented nearly every possible experience of violence to its audience, two specific instances stood out as remarkable during the course of gameplay. The first sequence featured the player interrogating and torturing a captured subject for reasons unknown to the player at the time of the course of actions. This torture sequence allowed the player to select their own torture devices, ranging from 'waterboarding' to electrocution. The torture victim was a man of ambiguous Middle Eastern ethnicity who spoke with a heavy accent. He repeatedly begged the player to stop during the sequence, yet the player could not advance in the game without torturing the victim with a minimum of three different devices. The second sequence involved an unprovoked spree of violence, disproportionate in reaction to the actions that preceded it. In this instance, the character being played was tasked to kill as many 'hipsters' as possible in a two-minute time period. This sequence occurred after the played character became offended by a predetermined interaction with a young man at a coffee shop who insulted the character's clothes. After the altercation, the played character entered what was referred to as a "Rampage Mission," and was given a monetary reward for both the number of people killed in this public space, and how quickly the player carried out the killings. During the course of this "Rampage Mission," the played character used weapons ranging from assault rifles, handguns, shotguns, explosive devices, and brass knuckles to kill pedestrians, all in a public shopping area. Game 1 was given a rating of M by the ESRB for "Blood and Gore, Intense Violence, Mature Humor, Nudity, Strong Language, Strong Sexual Content, [and] Use of Drugs and Alcohol" (ESRB, 2016). While the

ESRB rating and content descriptors represent much of the game's content, scenes such as those described above would not be revealed to the consumer based on such ratings alone.

The second and third games played offered a different style of violence from the first, focused mainly on massive multi-player online (MMO) play with incentivized killing of other online players. Both games were FPS and featured story modes and MMO modes. Since MMO play may qualitatively differ from the story mode in its additional content, both games were played in MMO modes to serve the intent of the study. Game 2 had a narrative of fantasy, but online play centered on human characters fighting against other human characters. Although characters were human, the characters faces and bodies were obscured with suits of armor, and online play did not involve any in-game vocalizations or communications between the characters. While the violence in Game 2 was not nearly as gratuitous and varied as that described in Game 1, the social context of online play incentivized efforts toward extreme violence. The online play consisted mainly of 12-minute sessions where players would be selected to teams with other online players, and the first team to earn 50 kills would win. Points were awarded to individual players for the amount of kills during the session. This provided motivation for individual players to kill other players as frequently as possible, driving a shared motivation for violence in the group as a whole. In Game 2, violence was carried out primarily with firearms, but explosives and hand-to-hand combat also were used. In addition to incentive within the session, players received awards in an out-of-session online profile for the manner in which they killed other players; awards of distinction were awarded for shots to the head, breaking the neck of another player, killing another player through blunt force to the head, use of explosives, and repeated use of certain firearms. Game 2 was rated T by the ESRB for content involving "Blood, Mild Language, [and] Violence," and while all three content descriptors were represented in gameplay, the implication of "violence" in the ESRB description did not capture the breadth of the game's content (ESRB, 2016).

The gameplay in Game 3 was similar to that of Game 2; Game 3 was an FPS, an MMO, and provided similar social and in-game incentives to kill as frequently and efficiently as possible. The narrative in Game 3 was much closer to a depiction of reality, with all human characters and with settings that resembled cities in South America, Eastern Europe, and the United States. Focus remained on online gameplay for reasons stated above, and online gameplay followed a similar format as that in Game 2. Online sessions consisted of players being selected into teams of eight players each, where the first team to earn 75 kills would win. Gameplay was markedly faster in Game 3, as most sessions would last about 6–10 minutes despite the higher number of kills needed to win. Players were awarded points for the number of players killed, as well as the manner in which they killed another player. Extra points were earned for shots to the head, killing a player with a knife, use of explosives, and repeated use of certain firearms. Unlike Game 2, Game 3 displayed much more blood and gore during its gameplay; "wounded" players would have blood displayed around the edges of their screens, other characters could be seen bleeding profusely, and blood spatter could be seen on walls and floors during gameplay. In addition, characters often did not have their faces obscured, unlike in Game 2. Both Game 2 and Game 3 displayed a violence that focused more on military-style efficiency and frequency. Social incentive through MMO play and in-game prompting motivated players to kill as many other players as possible, to frequently use certain firearms, and to carry out killings in brutal executions. Game 3 was given a rating of M by the ESRB for "Blood and Gore, Drug Reference, Intense Violence,

[and] Strong Language." While this rating represents much of the game's content, online incentives for such actions as stabbing other players or shooting other players in the head are not implied in the ESRB rating.

The fourth and fifth games were less violent than the first three games, yet maintained displays of blood and use of firearms. Neither game socially incentivized killing in the manner of Game 2 or Game 3, nor did Game 4 and Game 5 show in-game prompting for excessive and frequent violence. Game 4 was a MMORPG and an FPS, with more focus placed on the fantasy narrative and development of the character. While Game 4 did exhibit plenty of violence, most of the violence did not fall under our operational definition of unprovoked violence, as most of it came in self-defense. There were few instances in which the character was prompted to engage in unprovoked violence. Much of the gameplay centered on missions with nonviolent goals (i.e., recovery of items, traveling to meet other characters, discovery of new areas in the MMO game map). The social MMO component of Game 4 incentivized social interaction and trading of goods and services, unlike the socially incentivized violence exhibited in Games 2 and 3. When the played character did engage in unprovoked acts of violence, they involved assassination-style killings with the use of firearms resembling heavy caliber rifles. Other violence in the game, while not under the operational definition of unprovoked, used knives, explosives, and various firearms to attack nonhuman characters. Game 4 was given a rating of T for "Animated Blood, [and] Violence." This rating may be more representative than those given to Games 1, 2, and 3, yet descriptors of "animated blood" and "violence" are not sufficient in their implication of in-game violence and its consequences (ESRB, 2016).

Game 5 was similar to Game 4 in that most of the narrative sought to minimize violence when possible, and resulted in few instances of unprovoked violence. Game 5 alternated between FPS and TPS and was not an MMO. The thematic elements of Game 5 positioned the game as politically and militarily focused, with the played character acting as an agent of espionage in a reinterpretation of Cold War era global affairs. While the played character was explicitly capable and willing of violence, only a few acts of violence fell under our definition of unprovoked. Similar to Game 4, these instances resembled assassinations, and one instance involved the killing of a civilian by the played character. The executed civilian (a middle-aged man of ambiguous Hispanic descent) was wrongly assumed to be an enemy combatant due to skin color and an exaggerated accent. This victim, whose hands were bound behind his back, was shot in the back of the head with a pistol despite the victim's pleas to be spared. This content was similar to that seen in Game 1, where racial undertones were juxtaposed with an act of senseless and unprovoked violence. Political motivations and self-defense excluded many instances of violence from the operational definition of senseless or unprovoked violence, yet the game as a whole featured numerous violent encounters. The played character made use of knives, strangulation, explosives, nerve gas, and various firearms to defend against enemy combatants. Game 5 was given a rating of M by the ESRB for "Blood and Gore, Intense Violence, Sexual Themes, [and] Strong Language" (ESRB, 2016). These descriptors fit the much of the content of the game, yet do not adequately imply the content of such scenes as the execution of a civilian previously described.

The final game played featured the highest frequency and number of unprovoked violent acts, as the only objective in this fighter game was to kill the opponent in any manner possible. This game had no explicit narrative, and the characters varied from direct depictions of human men and women to persons taking a quasi-human form. Unlike the previous games,

Game 6 was not FPS or TPS, and was not an MMO. The camera angle of the game positioned the players as a third person audience to a close-quarters fight between the played character and one opponent. Due to the clear objective of the aforementioned violence, the time of each match varied in length from 4 to 12 minutes on average. During the course of the match, characters would mainly engage in hand-to-hand combat, although some characters employed knives and blunt objects to attack their opponent. In this game, nearly every action of a character was one of unprovoked violence under the operational definition; self-defense was not taken into consideration since the characters had no regard for self-preservation, and only sought to kill the opponent. Game 6 featured the most blood and gore out of any of the games played, with an excessive portrayal of blood for each injury sustained in the match. Particular violent acts elicited cut-scenes with detailed depictions of human viscera; such actions were incentivized due to the large damage inflicted on the opponent, and occurred frequently during gameplay. In these cut-scenes, images included, but were not limited to: slow-motion view of a character ripping the heart out of another character; depictions of a human spine being broken in half; and a depiction of a human skull being crushed. Game 6 proved to be an outlier in the sheer volume of violence depicted as well as the explicit nature of the game's intent. Game 6 was given a content rating of M by the ESRB for "Blood and Gore, Intense Violence, Strong Language," yet such descriptions of "blood and gore" and "intense violence" may not sufficiently imply the in-game acts of violence and their graphic representations (ESRB, 2016).

## Discussion

To date, there are no comprehensive published lists detailing the exact types of violent acts that players of certain video games may commit. The purpose of this study was to provide a detailed description of the senseless acts of violence in top-selling violent video games of the previous fiscal year. The study provides a novel description of video game violence, because it describes acts in later parts of games that have not been described previously. Since video games are the second least monitored media activity (Roberts, 1999), this study essentially monitored a handful of the top selling games so that consumers and players can have more detailed information about them. Parents who do monitor their children's media exposure tend to influence their children's understanding and reactions to game content (Gentile & Walsh, 2002) and, as a result, bringing knowledge to the public has the potential to change parenting practices related to VVG exposure.

Our study found that the ESRB rating system often did not fully portray the type of violence implied by their rating that was actually seen in game play. Much of the senseless violent content was only accessed through playing the games for significant periods of time. While some games were observed as less violent than others, the ratings for these games were still insufficient in their representation of content. While using the term "violence" (or the phrase "intense violence") in a content descriptor may represent some content of the game, rich information is lost when details such as torture, assassinations, mass shootings, ripping the heart out of another person, and crushing of human skulls are excluded. Although the warnings are on the package for "violence" and/or "strong language" in games rated "T for Teen," scenes of racism, torture, and added incentives for increased senseless violence were not described. It stands to reason that much of the public would question whether these themes are age appropriate for teenagers.

This study provides a high level of detail on the violent content of numerous video games. This may have important implications for consumers of these games, as well as for those who purchase these games for minors. For example, while the public may be aware that many current video games are violent in themes and content, much of the public may not realize that these games may involve, for example, killing large groups of people in public spaces with assault rifles, torturing people in a racially motivated context, detailed depictions of human viscera, and online social situations that incentivize frequent and efficient violence. By providing more precise content depictions, the results from this and similar studies may be used to improve parents' and consumers' media literacy. Many parents are mindful that the existing rating system does not provide all the information they want, are not accurate, and they often do not use it (Gentile et al., 2011). Detailed content descriptions of games would allow parents to more effectively determine what is appropriate for their child at any given age based on their personal preferences.

The extensive senseless violence seen in these five games is particularly concerning given the established link between violent video game use and desensitization to violence, aggressive thoughts and actions as well as affect (Nije, Konjin, & Bushman, 2012). If, as past research has suggested, VVGs "prime" players to conceive of violent acts they play in the game (Anderson, 2003), then players of these games may more readily conceive of mass shootings, race-related violence, assassination, and other themes.

This study has several limitations that are worthy of mention. First, it was not possible to fully play all of the violent games available on the market, leaving the content of many games unknown. Furthermore, the choices the players make during the game determine in part what content they will experience. For example, Game 1 allowed the player to engage in violent acts at their own discretion, leaving the possibility for the player to engage in minimal or even no acts of violence if they so choose. In addition, while it is possible that each of the two-hour playing sessions per game adequately represented the game content and experience, it was not possible to play each game to its entirety. Therefore, all of the acts of violence accessible in the games played may not have been discovered.

To better assess whether and how the violent content affects players, future studies should measure the player's and buyer's expectations of the games and compare those that to the actual violence observed. It would be useful, for example, to objectively measure players' reactions to unexpected violence (e.g., by tracking heart rate variability, skin conductance, self-report of feelings and thoughts) in games. Also, it may be useful to expose parents to game content and assess whether this affects their buying habits or limits set for their children.

In summary, the findings of this study can serve as meaningful insight into the kinds of problematic VVG content that are increasingly available to minors and suggest more thorough content descriptions in publicly accessible rating systems. Efforts should be made to significantly increase the public's understanding of the true content of VVGs. Lastly, parents and caregivers should be encouraged to use content rating systems and limit and monitor their children's game play.

# References

Abelman, R. (1990). Determinants of parental mediation of children's television viewing. In J. Bryant (Ed.), *Television and the American Family* (pp. 311–328). Hillsdale NJ: Lawrence Erlbaum and Associates.

Anderson, C. (2003). Violent video games: Myths, facts, and unanswered questions studies provide converging evidence that exposure to media violence is a significant risk factor for aggressive and violent behavior. *American Psychological Association Psychological Science Agenda: Science Briefs.* Retrieved February 28, 2016, from http://www.apa.org/science/about/psa/2003/10/anderson.aspx

Anderson, C., Shibuya, A., Ihori, N., Swing, E., Bushman, B., Sakamoto, A., ... & Saleem, M. (2010). Violent video game effects on aggression, empathy, and prosocial behavior in eastern and western countries: A meta-analytic review. *American Psychological Association Psychological Bulletin, 136,* 151–173.

Beasley, B., & Collins Standley, T. (2002). Shirts vs. skins: Clothing as an indicator of gender role stereotyping in video games. *Mass Communication & Society, 5,* 279–293.

Bijvank, M. N., Konijn, E. A., Bushman, B. J., & Roelofsma, P. H. (2009). Age and violent-content labels make video games forbidden fruits for youth. *Pediatrics, 123,* 870–876.

Brekke, A.D. (2006). Video game ratings: Does the system work for parents? (Unpublished master's thesis), The University of Tennessee Knoxville, Knoxville, Tennessee.

Bushman, B. J., & Anderson, C. A. (2002). Violent video games and hostile expectations: A test of the general aggression model. *Personality and social psychology bulletin, 28,* 1679–1686.

Bushman, B. J., & Huesmann, L. R. (2006). Short-term and long-term effects of violent media on aggression in children and adults. *Archives of Pediatrics & Adolescent Medicine, 160*(4), 348–352.

Calvert, C. (2002). Violence, video games, and a voice of reason: Judge Posner to the defense of kids' culture and the first amendment. *San Diego Law Review, 39,* 1.

Cantor, J. (1998). Ratings for program content: The role of research findings. *The Annals of the American Academy of Political and Social Science, 557,* 54–69.

Colón-de Martí, L. N., Rodríguez-Figueroa, L., Nazario, L. L., Gutiérrez, R., & González, A. (2011). Video games use patterns and parenteral supervision in a clinical sample of Hispanic adolescents 13–17 years old. *Boletin de la Asociacion Medica de Puerto Rico, 104,* 23–31.

Downs, E., & Smith, S. L. (2010). Keeping abreast of hypersexuality: A video game character content analysis. *Sex Roles, 62,* 721–733.

Entertainment Software Ratings Board (ESRB). (2016). *ESRB Ratings Guide.* Retrieved February 22, 2016, from http://www.esrb.org/ratings/ratings_guide.aspx

Gentile, D. (2009). Pathological video-game use among youth ages 8 to 18 a national study. *Psychological Science, 20,* 594–602.

Gentile, D. A., Maier, J. A., Hasson, M. R., de Bonetti, B. L. (2011). Parents' evaluation of media ratings a decade after the television ratings were introduced. *Pediatrics, 128*, 36–44. doi:10.1542/peds.2010-3026

Gentile, D. A., & Walsh, D. A. (2002). A normative study of family media habits. *Journal of Applied Developmental Psychology, 23*, 157–178.

Haninger, K., & Thompson, K. M. (2004). Content and ratings of teen-rated video games. *The Journal of the American Medical Association, 291*, 856–865.

Hartmann, T., Krakowiak, K. M., & Tsay-Vogel, M. (2014). How violent video games communicate violence: A literature review and content analysis of moral disengagement factors. *Communication Monographs, 81*, 310–332.

Ivory, A. H., & Kaestle, C. E. (2013). The effects of profanity in violent video games on players' hostile expectations, aggressive thoughts and feelings, and other responses. *Journal of Broadcasting & Electronic Media, 57*, 224–241.

Nije B. M., Konijn E. A., & Bushman B. J. (2012). "We don't need no education": Video game preferences, video game motivations, and aggressiveness among adolescent boys of different educational ability levels. *Journal of Adolescence, 35*, 153–162.

Oxford Dictionaries. (2016). *Definition of unprovoked in English*. Retrieved February 23, 2016, from http://www.oxforddictionaries.com/us/definition/american_english/unprovoked

Padilla-Walker, L. M., Nelson, L. J., Carroll, J. S., & Jensen, A. C. (2010). More than a just a game: Video game and internet use during emerging adulthood. *Journal of Youth and Adolescence, 39*, 103–113.

Ranj, B. (2016, May 02). *The 20 best-selling games of the last year*. Retrieved July 01, 2016, from http://www.businessinsider.com/best-selling-video-games-2015-2016-5

Reeves, T. D. (2009). Tort liability for manufacturers of violent video games: A situational discussion of the causation calamity. *Alabama Law Review, 60*, 519-546.

Rideout, V. J., Foehr, U., & Roberts, D. (2010). *Generation M 2—media in the lives of 8-to 18 year olds: A Kaiser Family Foundation study*. Retrieved February 21, 2016, from http://kff.org/other/event/generation-m2-media-in-the-lives-of/

Roberts, D. F. (1999). Kids & Media@ the New Millennium: A Kaiser Family Foundation Report. A Comprehensive National Analysis of Children's Media Use. Executive Summary.

Smith, S. L. (2006). *Perps, pimps, and provocative clothing: Examining negative content patterns in video games*. Retrieved February 20, 2016, from http://psycnet.apa.org/psycinfo/2006-05034-005

Strasburger, V. C., & Donnerstein, E. (1999). Children, adolescents, and the media: Issues and solutions. *Pediatrics, 103*, 129–139.

Thompson, K. M., Tepichin, K., & Haninger, K. (2006). Content and ratings of mature-rated video games. *Archives of Pediatrics & Adolescent Medicine, 160*, 402–410.

Walsh, D. A. (2000, March 21). *Interactive violence and children: Testimony submitted by the committee on commerce, science, and technology, United States senate*. Minneapolis, MN: National Institute on Media and the Family. Retrieved July 26, 2016, from https://www.gpo.gov/CHRG-106shrg7

Walsh, D. A., & Gentile, D. A. (2001). A validity test of movie, television, and video-game ratings. *Pediatrics, 107*, 1302–1308.

Weber R., Ritterfeld U., & Mathiak K. (2006). Does playing violent video games induce aggression? Empirical evidence of a functional magnetic resonance imaging study. *Media Psychology, 8*, 39–60.

# Making Sense of the Brutality of the Holocaust: Critical Themes and New Perspectives

Eric D. Miller

**ABSTRACT**

This article offers an analytic, integrative review of select themes associated with one of history's greatest atrocities: the Holocaust. Much of this review considers general and Holocaust-specific themes as they pertain to the nature of senseless violence and evil. The importance of having a greater understanding of the sheer brutality of violence perpetuated in the Holocaust is emphasized. As part of this discussion, considerable attention is given to how Internet-based photographs and videos from the Holocaust era can provide greater insight into understanding the evil associated with this genocide. Some consideration of the larger meaning of the Holocaust, particularly for Jews, is also examined.

The Holocaust can be an overwhelming area to examine for several academic and humanitarian reasons. Indeed, the Holocaust remains one of the darkest chapters in all of human history. The Holocaust as an event in human history demands an extensive examination of how it came to be, from historic roots of European anti-Semitism to Hitler's rise to power and his aggressive, virulent and racist agenda to invasions of countries featuring mass segregation of Jewish populations to decisions to enact full-scale genocide. The Holocaust continues to be examined today not just from a historical lens but also from a broader social scientific and psychological perspective. Considerable research and scholarship has attempted to answer how individuals en masse could either wantonly or indirectly allow for the slaughter of millions of men, women, and children on account of their religious and ethnic identity. When we consider the atrocities committed during the Holocaust era, it is important to remember that millions of non-Jews were also murdered by the Nazis and their perpetrators. Naturally, these deaths are no less grievous than the ones committed against the Jews. However, this article aims to focus on the group that was unquestionably the focus of Nazi genocidal policies: the Jews (including the widely recognized failure to help European Jews during the Holocaust). In considering this topic, it is also important to add that the study of the Holocaust can almost seem like an unbearable topic to consider because it is illustrative of profoundly egregious human cruelty and suffering that will likely forever haunt the conscience of humanity.

This article first offers some general considerations and definitions of senseless violence with particular emphasis on the nature of the brutality displayed against Jews during the Holocaust. The latter goal is accomplished with an interdisciplinary analysis of psychological, historical, journalistic, and other social science sources. As is discussed in this article, a clear challenge for psychologists and social scientists has been to define precisely what constitutes "evil" behavior in the context of senseless violence. A particularly unique contribution of this article is its discussion of the value of online Holocaust imagery (such as photographic and video evidence from that era) in both a general sense and, specifically, to allow for a greater potential understanding of the social psychological roots of evil. Another critical aspect of this special issue is the consideration of how individuals and society-at-large tries to come to terms with senseless violence. In that respect, this article next explores some central themes in how Holocaust survivors (and their offspring) and the Jewish people (more generally) have tried to make sense of this cataclysmic genocide. In totality, these critical themes are so highlighted in that they may offer an important perspective on the meaning of senseless violence.

## Recognizing and Defining Senseless Violence and Evil: General Considerations and its Relevance to the Holocaust

In some respects, defining senseless violence of any sort should almost seem like a very straight-forward proposition. Indeed, Lodewijkx, Wildschut, Nijstad, Savenije, and Smit (2001) offer experimental evidence that individuals are more apt to label senseless violence as such when a hypothetical victim is not blamed or involved with a given perpetrator; by doing so, these and other researchers (e.g., Van Zomeren & Lodewijkx, 2005) suggest that such views help to provide some semblance of a belief in a just world (e.g., Lerner, 1980). However, Duck (2009) cautions that behavior, such as murder, that the public would generally view as senseless or random violence is often not perceived that way by those who commit such acts; as an example, he notes that those involved with drug gang violence often consider "acts of murder…to be closely tied to local orders of expectation and practice" (p. 419).

Some of this controversy may be complicated by the point that some can argue about who is a "victim" and a "perpetrator." From the perspective of an assumed perpetrator, such as a Nazi, he or she may not have necessarily viewed his or her actions as injurious and, in fact, they may have been perceived as being well justified (Baumeister, 1999). As Hannah Arendt (1963) famously concluded from the 1961 trial of Adolf Eichmann, many Nazis felt that they simply were akin to cogs in a machine where they followed orders from presupposed leaders. In fact, Arendt's analysis of a so-called "banality of evil" had some impact on the classic work of social psychologist Stanley Milgram's (1963, 1974) famous studies of obedience. While still acknowledging the tremendous impact that his work continues to have on the field, Milgram's methods and conclusions have been severely criticized on many grounds (e.g., Reicher, Haslam, & Miller, 2014). Even those who have largely praised the work of Milgram (e.g., Blass, 1998), while admitting some general linkages between Milgram's work and understanding the Holocaust, there has been an appreciation for its limitations as well:

> …Milgram's approach does not provide a fully adequate explanation of the Holocaust. While it may well account for the dutiful destructiveness of the dispassionate bureaucrat who may have

shipped Jews to Auschwitz with the same degree of routinization as potatoes to Bremenhaven, it falls short when one tries to apply it to the more zealous, inventive, and hate-driven atrocities that also characterized the Holocaust. (p. 51)

Consistent with the aforesaid statement, distinguished social psychologist Leonard Berkowitz (1999)—using some of Arendt's own words—makes the point that evil, particularly with respect to the atrocities committed during the Holocaust, cannot be simply viewed as banal behavior:

> No one had issued orders that infants should be thrown into the air as shooting targets, or hurled into the fire alive, or have their heads smashed against walls....Innumerable individual crimes, one more horrible than the next, surrounded and created the atmosphere of the gigantic crime of extermination. (Arendt, as cited in Berkowitz, 1999, p. 250)

Arthur Miller (2014) further suggests that social psychology may be guilty of "glossing over the gratuitous brutality of the Holocaust...[in favor of focusing on a] preoccupation with the Milgram experiments" (p. 566). This brutality is indeed not pleasant to dwell upon but it is critical to emphasize the Holocaust's multi-faceted aspects of cruelty, deception, and murder. *The Holocaust Chronicle* (Harran, Kuntz, Lemmons, Michael, Pickus, Roth, & Edelheit, 2000), among other sources, provides an extensive documentation of many of these many cruelties from (and even predating) Hitler's rise to power in 1933 until the end of World War II in 1945 (and shortly thereafter). Some of these atrocities include (but certainly are not limited to): segregation of Jews from the larger society, the removal of all of one's personal belongings, the forcible displacement and starvation of Jews in ghettos, constant humiliation and degrading behaviors (e.g, washing streets) to the ultimate "Final Solution" of mass genocide (Harran et al., 2000). As unpleasant as it is to consider, even the methods of death for the Jews and others varied considerably. For instance, *Einsatzgruppen* consisted of Nazi SS guards and local authorities, who gunned down entire Jewish populations within towns largely in Eastern Europe. Even though Auschwitz remains arguably the best known Concentration Camp, Nazis experimented with various methods of killing, such as gas vans at the Chelmno Concentration Camp, long before the mass manufacturing of genocide took place at the aforementioned site. Not only did Jews commonly have to pay for their own tickets under the guise of relocation but elaborate schemes (such as the construction of fake ticket/train stations) were concocted and devised in order to hide the true plans of the Nazis. To add to the perversity of this violence, some Jews (selected as *Sonderkommandos*) were even forced to aid the Nazis with the execution and aftermath of mass killings of fellow Jews only to be murdered later. Even with imminent Nazi defeat, Jews—already greatly suffering from Concentration Camp imprisonment—were commonly forced to go on "Death Marches." Those who ultimately survived often waited for very uncertain futures as displaced persons—and, in some cases, still faced violence (or death) even if they attempted to return to their original hometowns. Opotow (2011) summarizes many of the antecedental acts that allowed for the Holocaust as being a form of extreme moral exclusion where concerns for fairness, sharing resources, and well-being of others are largely absent; some acts included exclusion within society (e.g., barred from professions, forcible relocation), exclusion from society (e.g., forcible deportation, slave labor), and exclusion as annihilation (e.g., starvation and murder). Recent research from the United States Holocaust Museum has buttressed the point that the Holocaust was not an act of isolated violence but rather mass murder that truly encompassed most of Nazi-occupied Europe: It is now estimated that over 42,500 Nazi ghettos, slave labor sites, and concentration camps—significantly more than previously believed—were in operation between 1933 and 1945 across Europe (Lichtblau, 2013).

The question of how and why the Holocaust occurred and why the Jews, in particular, were targeted is an incredibly complex issue. To offer a rather cursory explanation, McMillan (2014) suggests that Jews were a target across Europe because they were, in fact, living all across Europe. That is, because they were a minority across all of Europe, it was relatively easy to demonize Jews on account of their non-Christianity, perceived or fabricated sense of otherness, envy of success of select Jews, and alleged questionable political alliances and allegiances. McMillan (2014) adds though what may have been particularly virulent to German anti-Semitism was a belief that "the Jewish people constituted a *race* that was biologically distinct from the rest of all humanity and genetically predisposed to behave destructively" (p. 152). A related Nazi construct was *Lebensraum* (or "living space") where Hitler decreed that Germany had a right and need to physically expand to meet its own needs for their own people; inherent in this ideology would be the removal of those from these lands who were not of 'German blood' per the dictates of Nazi ideology. Other scholars add that many of the early acts that Germans took against the Jews (such as *Kristallnacht*, or "The Night of Broken Glass") largely echoed previous acts of mob violence, or pogroms, taken against the Jews largely throughout their existence on the European continent; however, the sheer methods of killing on a mass scale (e.g., Bronner, 1999) and the indifference or inaction by many parties during the killings (such as the allies, including America, other European countries and citizenry, and the clergy; Fettweis, 2003) adds to this devastating historic record of genocide.

Many academics and non-academics alike have wrestled with the broader meaning of "evil." Social psychologist Philip Zimbardo (2004), the author of the classic Stanford Prison Study, suggests that "Evil is intentionally behaving –or causing others to act – in ways that demean, dehumanize, harm, destroy, or kill innocent people" (p. 23). Another esteemed social psychologist, Ervin Staub (1989, 1999, 2014) has outlined the basic conditions that allow for (or have allowed for) expressions of evil particularly in the context of genocide and the Holocaust. In short, Staub suggests that a conglomeration of social, cultural, and personal factors can foment evil including a desire to fulfill basic or personal needs, a desire for collective action (even if it is destructive towards others), a changing or acceptance of deviant norms, high respect and desire for authority, and bystander passivity. Haslam and Reicher (2007) add that perpetrators, or those who would harm (or encourage harm to others) typically do so with conviction and those who might adhere to destructive ideologies are particularly likely to possess certain personal-based qualities (such as social dominance and aggressive tendencies); once drawn to such ideology, consistent with the dynamics of group membership, such individuals often feel a greater investment in these groups and a potential desire to recruit others to the cause.

To offer a slightly different perspective, Berkowitz (1999) argues that "evil" should be thought of as a concept where there are certain differential grades of evil. With a consideration of the Holocaust as a backdrop, Berkowitz states: "Some acts are more evil than others. Thus, we might consider the brutal killing of a young child to be evil because our conception of this event resembles our prototype of evil but not think of a husband's beating his wife as very evil because our understanding of this battering is far removed from this prototype" (p. 251). However, he concedes that evil may be construed as a somewhat fuzzy concept and that individuals may have varying ideas as to what constitutes evil. While more research should aim to flesh out these points, Berkowitz adds that: "for many people, the actions and policies we usually associate with Hitler have a close resemblance to their prototype of evil" (p. 251).

Berkowitz (1999) also makes it clear that he is not necessarily nominating the Holocaust, as the "most" evil event of all time. In fact, in addressing his focus on the mass killing of European Jews during the Holocaust, he expressly states: "This focus certainly does not mean that I believe the Nazis' killing of Gypsies, homosexuals, and seriously handicapped persons was necessarily less evil than the Holocaust, or that Stalin or Pol Pot (or any others one might nominate) were not evil" (p. 252). And yet, his perspective forces us to consider that people may indeed view certain events as "evil"—however, depending on the situational context of these events or how certain events are juxtaposed, some "evil" acts may seem not quite as "evil" in relation to another event. For instance, in this formulation, the terrorist attacks of September 11, 2001 are widely acknowledged as being the single-most photographed and videoed war-related event in history and, arguably, the suffering inflicted upon thousands on that day would meet the criteria of what is evil. However, perhaps consistent with this logic, the events of 9/11—while still illustrating evil—may seem not quite as "evil" in comparison to sheer extent of devastating and devious behavior (including the loss of life) accompanying the Holocaust.

Consistent with the aforesaid argument, the case could be made that even in comparison to other genocides different gradients of evil could be considered. While a natural concern might be that such an analysis could be used to minimize or deny suffering (which surely should be avoided), such comparisons can serve to provide a different understanding of the qualities of evil. In fact, Flanzbaum (1999) notes that in American culture, the horrors of the Holocaust were far from being emphasized—or even fully known—in the immediate decades following the Holocaust. She notes that, for decades, Americans' knowledge of the Holocaust largely came from the relatively benign early publications of *The Diary of Anne Frank* which downplayed the horrors of this genocide; in later decades, with increased awareness of these horrors through both survivor accounts and high profile public events (such as the opening of the U.S. Holocaust Museum and the release of the 1993 film *Schindler's List*), the American public began to appreciate these horrors from a deeper perspective.

A complicating factor in trying to consider meaningful analyses of different genocide-related events is that some scholars have argued over the precise meaning of an act of genocide (including from a legal sense). For instance, Schabas (2000) contends that though the acts of the Khmer Rouge in Cambodia in the late 1970s and the Milosevic forces in Kosovo in 1999 should be viewed as atrocities they should not necessarily be viewed as acts of genocide. In discussing the atrocities of Pol Pot's Khmer Rouge, he suggests that these victims were largely identified by their social and economic standing—and not the intentional destruction of a national, religious, racial, or ethnic group as called for according to the legal definition of genocide in the 1948 Convention on the Prevention and Punishment of the Crime of Genocide. Regarding the Kosovo conflicts, he argues for the importance of distinguishing genocide from ethnic cleaning such that the latter "generally involves killing, but with the intent to effect forced migration from a territory" (p. 295). With genocide, as shown in the Holocaust, mass murder is the ultimate goal.

Other scholars have made the case that the Holocaust represented a particularly unique and insidious form of genocide. For example, Heinsohn (2000) argues that Hitler's (and the Third Reich's) obsession against the Jews is fairly well-known, including the point that this genocide was viewed as having a higher importance than the general war effort. However, he contends that the Holocaust was not just a means to murder all Jews, but it was also a potential means to encourage and justify all future acts of genocide (to have been committed by the Nazis) after removing Judaism's principles surrounding the sanctity of life from German society. Moshman (2001) offers many paradoxical views about how to conceptualize genocide vis-à-vis the Holocaust, such as: the Holocaust receives incredible attention yet its focus is clearly justified, the Holocaust obviously is a prototypical case of genocide yet its focus confuses our understanding of other acts of genocide, and while genocide is often appropriately viewed as the ultimate act of evil, it is inaccurate to assume that a non-genocidal event cannot also be evil. He suggests that "The Holocaust is both worse than we can ever imagine as well as a small part of a larger picture" (p. 448) of violations of human rights.

Friedrichs (2000) puts forth the somewhat conflicting notion that even if the Holocaust may not necessarily be the most evil event of all-time (though it may be), it nonetheless encompassed a truly grotesque form of violence. On one hand, he contends that: "No claim is made here, then, that the Holocaust was necessarily the worst case of genocide in history. Indeed, some have argued that other cases of genocide—for example, the genocide directed at Native Americans—were more enduring and resulted in much greater loss of life [and b]y some estimations, more people died in Mao's People's Republic of China...Is it really possible (or desirable) to have a comparative sociology of cruelty, or relative evil?" (p. 22). And yet, not only does he suggest that the Holocaust profoundly shaped Jewish and world history (in part, by giving a clear definition of genocide), but he contends it is effectively the "crime of the century" for showcasing how individuals, groups, nations, and governmental entities could (at so many vast levels) ensure the mass mistreatment, destruction, and ultimate murder of a group of individuals on account of their race or religion.

Friedrichs (2000) also offers some insightful comments as how to best understand and categorize evil. He suggests that homicides (and other crimes) are often viewed differently than genocides. Indeed, Welner's (2009) Depravity Scale, a well-known measure of criminal evil, tends to focus on personal characteristics that make one predisposed to carry out violent crimes. Though he does not explicitly acknowledge this point, Friedrichs (2000) appears sympathetic to the idea that man-made mass causality events may particularly embody evil. For instance, in trying to imagine what the "crime of the century" may be when looking back from the year 2100, he suggests: "Arguably the single most disturbing possibility is a nuclear holocaust with a scope almost unimaginable to us" (p. 34).

In considering the totality of this analysis, it appears that certain factors may help to define an event as especially evil: greater loss of life, the methods used to cause death (including the degree to which others have conspired to produce it), death caused exclusively due to personal-based characteristics including (but not limited to) race, religion, ethnicity, or gender, and deaths committed against children. Clearly, the Holocaust contained all of these qualities. Future research should aim to clarify and quantify how individuals make distinctions about historic events (e.g., the Holocaust, the Cambodian atrocities, and 9/11) regarding their relative degree of evil as well as the more abstract characteristics of what constitutes evil behavior and actions. Such research may have the practical effect of allowing for greater awareness of past injustices as well as the hope for the prevention of future atrocities.

## Utilizing Online Imagery to Study The Senseless Violence and Evil of the Holocaust

Hungarian film director László Nemes received much acclaim for his 2015 award- winning motion picture "Son of Saul." Nemes suggested that people today still have not fully acknowledged the trauma of the Holocaust and may not necessarily be able to do so without having a full visual appreciation of it. To that end, he stated: "Since the end of the Second World War I've seen very clearly that many people more or less consider the Holocaust as a mythical story and approached it probably from a defensive mechanism, as a way to get away from it through survival stories…I don't think Auschwitz and the extermination of the European Jews was about survival. It was about death. And how Europe killed itself, committed suicide… This generation, the next generations need to be presented with the visual experience that brings them back to the here and now of the concentration camp and have the point of view in the story applied to one human being" (Donadio, 2015, p. 2).

Nemes clearly argues not just for a more fuller acknowledgment of the widespread brutality perpetrated against the Jews of Europe in the 1930s and 1940s but also makes the case that visual images can and should be used as a means to depict the nature of this brutality. Indeed, the availability of photographic evidence of mass trauma and wartime carnage available for the larger public predates the Holocaust by almost a century. Photographer Alexander Gardner is widely credited for providing the first images of wartime during the 1862 Battle of Antietam that took place near Sharpsburg, Maryland; this critical Civil War battle is particularly notorious for being equated with the single-most bloodiest day in American history to date where over 3,600 soldiers were killed and thousands more were injured or went missing. Gardner's photographs of Antietam, which were displayed in New York City, were critical in showing to the public that war should not be viewed as something that is glamorous but rather as an event that showcases war's pure butchery (E. D. Miller, 2011).

To forge ahead some 80 years or so to the timeframe of the Holocaust, numerous photographic and even video evidence was taken to showcase and depict Nazi Germany's war against the Jews. Indeed, much of the select photographic evidence that does exist were taken by Nazis themselves—some of which was purportedly to be used for Hitler's twisted idea and notion of a "Museum of the Extinct Race" had they been ultimately victorious in World War II (Pavlát, 2008). Holocaust photography though did have a sort of unique historical duality though. Consistent with Hitler's purposeful decision to not formally visit Concentration Camps, only select archival footage was taken at Auschwitz—the most well-known death camp (Kershaw, 2005).

While select news and images of the Holocaust were available during the killings, in the decades following the Holocaust, a growing body of scholarship has noted that both the Roosevelt administration (e.g., Wyman, 1984) and newspaper organizations (such as *The New York Times*; Leff, 2005) tended to actively discount or downplay these events. In brief, regarding the former point, many historians (e.g., Beir & Josepher, 2013) point to the fact that not only were strict immigrant quotas not expanded; many spots that should have been theoretically available to European Jews remained unfilled (perhaps, in part, due to the anti-Semitic views of Roosevelt's Assistant Secretary of State Breckinridge Long who did not want to ensure that these quotas were maximized). One of the more infamous examples of Roosevelt's apparent indifference to Jewish refugees occurred when in 1939 over 900 German Jews left on a chartered boat (the *St. Louis*, which was initially headed to Cuba and ultimately denied entry there) and unsuccessfully tried to gain admittance to the United States (where all were forced to return to Europe and at least a quarter of them were eventually murdered in the Holocaust). Beir and Josepher add that another ongoing debate is the question over why the Roosevelt administration did not more aggressively attack or bomb the death camps like Auschwitz. Although these historical debates remain, they conclude that—given the historical climate at that time—Roosevelt should be commended for realizing the threat of Nazi Germany and believed that the best method of saving European Jews was to win the war. They add that not only did Roosevelt enjoy wide support from the American Jewish community at that time but many foes—both domestic and foreign—viewed Roosevelt as sympathetic to Jewish causes. Indeed, although it certainly does not justify the lack of forceful action to help European Jews seeking refuge in the United States at the time, it is important to note that the pre-Civil Rights World War II era was marked by many xenophobic, anti-Semitic, and racist attitudes (perhaps exacerbated by the years of the Great Depression) such that large majorities of Americans did not support the loosening of immigration quotas to European Jewish refugees (and perhaps not unlike the Syrian refugee crisis of today; Zeitz, 2015). If anything, Beir and Josepher, like Leff (2005), seem to heap more culpability toward newspaper organizations, particularly *The New York Times*, for downplaying the atrocities of the Holocaust. They state:

> The media kept Holocaust stories off the front pages. *The New York Times*, for instance, from the years 1939 through 1945, printed 1,186 Holocaust stories, or an average of 17 stories per month. And yet only 26 stories mentioning the 'discrimination, deportation, and destruction' of the Jews made the front pages. And of those stories, only six identified Jews as the primary victims. Six stories in 6 years. Six stories while six million died. (pp. 269–270)

Curiously, the then-owner of *The New York Times*, Arthur Sulzberger, was Jewish; Sulzberger may have tacitly allowed for this minimal reporting due to his own views of Jews and Judaism and out of concern for not seeming impartial to the larger public (Leff, 2006). As another fascinating example as to the potential power of Internet-based archival materials, in April 2016, the United States Holocaust Memorial Museum launched an ambitious call for all citizens to search for and submit all Holocaust-related reports from local American newspapers during 1933 to 1945; this project, "History Unfolded" aims to shed additional light on what was reported and what Americans may have known about the Holocaust from that time (Hamill, 2016). The ability to cull through these records electronically will likely make this endeavor more feasible to successfully accomplish.

Once the Camps were ultimately liberated by Americans and the allies, there is also evidence that some Holocaust-related footage was even purposely suppressed after the war. A particularly prominent example of this was the footage delivered as part of Alfred Hitchcock's powerful documentary "German Concentration Camps Factual Survey," which showed the horrific aftermath of the Holocaust along with the extensive existence of Concentration Camps across Nazi-occupied Europe; with the recent 2014 documentary "Night Will Fall," the story behind this film—including the decision to shelve it for fear of alienating Germany as a potential political ally following the war—was told (Hale, 2015).

An important question is what is new or different about *online* Holocaust imagery? First, and probably most obviously, with the Internet such imagery is no longer difficult to find and can be presented in unique and meaningful ways to a larger population. There are many Websites—such as those affiliated with Museums like the U.S. Holocaust Memorial Museum and Israel's Yad Vashem and other sites like "Jewish Virtual Library"—that house thousands of pictures showing the plight of European Jews before, during, and immediately after the Holocaust. One can also very easily utilize Google Images or visit other online/social media sites or groups to find countless photographs as well. In fact, on January 27, 2015, as part of the commemoration of the 70th anniversary of the liberation of the Auschwitz

Concentration Camp, Google organized an extensive online exhibition detailing several facets about the Holocaust.

One might also want to consider what could we want to do with such images and why would we want to engage with them? Naturally, by having an awareness of these images, we inherently offer an act of critical remembrance. After all, in his classic work *Night*, Holocaust survivor and Nobel Peace Prize winner Elie Wiesel (1958/2006) famously stated "To forget the dead would be akin to killing them a second time." To that point, Rassin, Rootselaar, Heiden, Ugahary, and Wagener (2005) demonstrated with experimental methods that those who could not clearly imagine World War II images—including those associated with the Holocaust—were more inclined to endorse beliefs indicative of exaggerations of Nazi cruelties.

Prior to the past decade or so, if one wanted to seek Holocaust footage, one had to actively seek it (e.g., in libraries) or perhaps found it difficult to fully comprehend and digest (e.g., in a school setting). With such online imagery, one can study, observe, and share these images at one's own choosing and perhaps with others. In doing so, we can even imagine (or try to imagine) the plight of those pictured in these images. Arguably, some of the most haunting and distressing images do not necessarily involve images of grotesque brutality; and, indeed, may feature images of over the one million children murdered in the Holocaust. One such example are pictures of the children who were placed in hiding at an orphanage in the southeastern hamlet of Izieu, France; a number of these photographs show these children appearing to be relatively content and enjoying the spoils of childhood despite the dire conditions of genocide and war lurking nearby. Any semblance of tranquility for these 42 children (and 5 of their caregivers) ended on April 6, 1944 when Nazi troops—led by the leading Gestapo officer Klaus Barbie—raided the orphanage and forcibly loaded the children onto trucks that would ultimately take all of them to their deaths at Auschwitz or other death camps (Klarsfeld, 1985).

Film from this era also can produce a similar effect of allowing us to try to fathom the losses that occurred while also trying to provide us with a semblance of understanding regarding the incredible suffering that was endured during this time. For instance, the documentary "Jewish Life in Bialystok" shows the proud day-to-day happenings of the Jewish community in Bialystok, Poland as it existed in the summer of 1939, which was literally weeks before the Nazi invasion of Poland. One can only surmise that most of those pictured in that film, like the social world depicted, simply vanished. But, it need not always be the case that European Jews pictured or filmed from the Holocaust era be forever unknown. Indeed, such media can even serve to answer some gaps in the historical record about the Holocaust as was accomplished with the release of Glenn Kurtz's, 2014 book and related short film "Three Minutes in Poland." In brief, while helping his parents clear out some personal belongings, Glenn Kurtz stumbled upon 70-year-old footage of his grandparents' visit to their ancestral towns near Warsaw, Poland in the summer of 1938. Kurtz's grandparents used a home video recorder that taped roughly 3 minutes of footage of a town that was decimated in the Holocaust. Upon realizing the importance of this film as a historical record of Polish Jewish life right before the onset of World War II and Holocaust, Kurtz worked with the U.S. Holocaust Memorial Museum to refurbish the film that was ultimately placed on its Website. A couple of years later, Kurtz received contacts suggesting that the identity of one of the individuals pictured in the film—a 13-year-old at the time—was positively identified by the granddaughter of this aforesaid individual. Amazingly, this individual, Morris Chandler was not just identified but also found living in the United States.

This case highlights that, particularly given the wide reach and availability of the Internet, the ability to further analyze and glean new information about the Holocaust—including about survivors and victims—still is quite possible. More generally, not only is there sometimes new information to be discovered about the Holocaust, but the potential for both academics and non-academics to gather new insights increases when historical archives and artifacts are placed online. For instance, the German organization The International Tracing Service—which houses over 30 million documents related to the Holocaust and Nazi persecution—recently began to publish its first 50,000 documents online. International Tracing Service archive department head Christian Groh aptly summarizes the importance of doing this by noting that: "Archives must not hide themselves from the digital world. Otherwise, one day they will be forgotten" ("Holocaust-era archive uploads," 2015, p. 1)

Not only can widespread availability of this imagery online provide the potential to greater educate the public about the history and trauma associated with the Holocaust, it may also help to provide greater insight into what precisely constitutes "evil." The use of such publicly available, archival sources may be particularly valuable given the inherent challenges of studying evil in terms of ethical and logistical constraints (e.g., Darley, 1999). Indeed, there is evidence that individuals can differentiate the underlying content found within traumatic events in an online context. For instance, an innovative content analysis of over 2,000 YouTube comments from four different YouTube videos related to the 2012 Sandy Hook Elementary School and Aurora theater mass shootings and the catastrophic Hurricane Sandy showed that YouTube comments associated with the Sandy Hook shootings (particularly those from a memorial video) were especially likely to feature compassion and grief with lessened hostility. Given these results, this study highlighted that even in an online environment, powerful situational contexts greatly guide behavior, such as how individuals show grief and related emotions following man-made and natural calamities (E. D. Miller, 2015). Accordingly, it bears to reason that online comments could likewise be able to make similar differentiations amongst different events, including those featuring Holocaust imagery.

However, there may be some challenges to using online Holocaust imagery as a means to study senseless violence and evil. Consider the tragic case and photograph of three year-old Aylan Kurdi: A photograph of Aylan's lifeless body on a Turkish beach was shown throughout the world (in September 2015) as it was believed to embody the Syrian refugee crisis, which is believed to be the one of the most serious humanitarian crisis since the end of World War II and the Holocaust (e.g., Peralta, 2014). To be clear, Aylan's death is incredibly heartbreaking, and the picture of his death makes this point all the more. However, if evil is to be conceptualized in different grades (e.g., Berkowitz, 1999), there is a risk that we could (however inadvertent) minimize suffering. As noted earlier, the deaths of over 1 million children may be one of the most horrifying qualities of the Holocaust. By acknowledging this point, does this somehow minimize the tragedy of the death of one child, such as Aylan? Yet, we can also look at this issue from the opposite perspective. Given how horrific the death of one child is, should it not make the deaths of over a million children in the Holocaust all the more horrific? This question also raises the provocative consideration about the power of social media—and what if it would have existed during World War II. Avi Benlolo, president of Canada's Friends of Simon Wiesenthal Center for Holocaust Studies suggests that it may have been used for the good. He suggests: "Had the digital age existed and had enough individuals been encouraged by mass social activism, one hopes the outcome would have been different" (Benlolo, 2012, p. 1).

Naturally, we can hope that would have been so; however, social media postings are sometimes known for their less than gracious comments. This brings another critical potential pitfall of the widespread availability of online Holocaust imagery: The ability of individuals to exploit such content as a means to denigrate the Holocaust and its victims or survivors. Moor, Heuvelman, and Verleur (2010) suggest that there are three major reasons why flaming (or extremely hostile or offensive language) may occur in social media, such as YouTube: (a) When we are online, we have a changed awareness of the self, including a perception of anonymity; (b) The prevalence of miscommunication and misunderstandings of both online material and conversations; and (c) An intentional act to state one's views online, particularly if they are views that might not be readily acceptable to overtly acknowledge in face-to-face communication. Regardless of the motivation, Moor et al. (2010) also found that while most of their sample did not report engaging in flaming, most have indeed witnessed it online. One could argue that those who would disparage or deny the suffering from the Holocaust merely represent a fringe view. Yet, in the case of Adolf Hitler's ideology, as highlighted throughout this article, both history and psychology have shown that even fringe views can reach a larger consensus under certain conditions. In a free and democratic society, ultimately, we may have to accept that the ability to abuse or misuse such images is a distinct possibility, although strident attempts can and should be undertaken to rally against such hateful expressions.

As noted earlier, online Holocaust imagery has the potential to allow researchers to better conceptualize the nature of evil and senseless violence both by studying the acts committed in archival footage and how individuals respond to such imagery (often in an online context). While Holocaust-era traditional photographs and related media still have the potential to convey powerful messages, there is growing evidence that individuals are increasingly utilizing online social imagery as a means to understand their sense of self (e.g., Davies, 2007). As such, there is the potential for individuals to draw more meaningful connections, insights, and compassion with regards to these images in an online format. A related set of questions might be whether it should be assumed that such images will necessarily produce a meaningful and positive effect in an individual and what fundamental purposes do these images even serve? Although greater research should further flesh out individual reasons for viewing such materials and their net effects on individuals, it is prudent to presume that there would likely be much variation in how individuals process such images. For instance, even among Jews, Wohl and Van Bavel (2011) found that post-traumatic symptoms were negatively correlated with having non-Holocaust descendants yet these symptoms were positively correlated with having Holocaust descendants (though these effects were lessened by the willingness of family members to discuss past family Holocaust-related history). Accordingly, consistent with the findings from the aforementioned study, a Jewish individual with Holocaust descendants might show heightened distress after viewing such imagery whereas a Jewish individual without such a family history might consider such imagery as a reminder of their proud collective identity.

The question of what is the fundamental purpose of Holocaust images and how they may differ from other traumatic images is arguably a much more challenging question to answer. Many have highlighted that Holocaust imagery may contain violent, traumatic injury but they also provide the viewer with a foreboding quality insomuch that we often imagine the victimization that the individual was experiencing in the image and would have likely experienced at a later point (including death). For instance, in contrasting Holocaust imagery with

9/11 imagery, Orbán (2007) suggests that while 9/11 images tend to be more focused on the immediate destruction of life (such as through the plane crashes and the tower collapses),

> Holocaust images overwhelmingly capture a prolonged approach or aftermath (such as images of people known in retrospect to have died shortly after having been photographed or images of what was found upon liberation of the concentration camps), thereby arguably further emphasizing the void between approach and aftermath. (p. 59)

Łysak (2016) makes not only a similar point insomuch that imagery from the Warsaw Ghetto has a haunting quality in that those depicted were not only suffering at the time but were (in most cases) subsequently murdered but also regarding the point about how we view and understand such imagery can change over time. After all, the Nazis who filmed these images were doing so for propaganda-based reasons consistent with their anti-Semitic agenda; now, such images serve as testimony to wanton misery. In considering lynching photographs, largely of African-Americans from the Jim Crow era of American history, Campbell (2004) likewise notes how these images largely conveyed different messages at the time they were taken versus how they are viewed now in that these photographs "were produced as celebratory icons of white supremacy, but are now read as powerful evidence of a deplorable racist history" (p. 71). He adds that while such images can be incredibly difficult to view, it is important to be mindful that many of these images were instrumental in helping to raise awareness and change attitudes; a particularly potent example was the purposeful decision of Emmet Till's mother to have her teenage son's mangled body widely photographed after he was lynched in 1955 for supposedly showing interest in a white woman in Mississippi. Campbell (2004) adds that in terms of presenting violent historical imagery there is a dual concern that oversaturation can lead viewers to perhaps feeling overwhelmed or even fatigued by such imagery and, yet, there is a grave danger to completely trying to hide away such images (particularly in terms of how they are represented in the media). Ultimately, he suggests that:

> …images do bring a particular kind of power to the portrayal of death and violence. Seeing the body and what has been done to it is important. Images alone might not be responsible for a narrative's power, but narratives that are un-illustrated can struggle to convey the horror evident in many circumstances. (p. 71)

The question of whether an image from the Holocaust, 9/11, or a lynching is more horrifying to view (and for whom), and its larger psychological effects on an individual, largely returns us to the earlier discussion on the nature of evil and how to possibly codify and compare differing events.

## Making Sense of the Holocaust

In the years since the Holocaust, many writings and accounts have been offered—by survivors and non-survivors alike—as to how both Jews and society-at-large can make sense of the horrors of the *Shoah*. Frankl's (1959) highly celebrated "Man's Search for Meaning" offers both insight into his own psychological experience as a Concentration Camp survivor but also his theories on the importance of searching for meaning in life; his analysis remains a particularly optimistic and hopeful suggestion that meaning can be found (and should be sought) even in the darkest of conditions. However, much of the subsequent literature and related accounts has found that survivors often have spoken of deep, personal pain related to their experiences during the Holocaust (e.g., Langer, 1991). The broad notion that Holocaust survivors, in comparison to peers who did not endure the Holocaust, have faced profound challenges to their psychological adjustment has been well-documented in the research literature; though such survivors frequently exhibit psychological resilience they also tend to exhibit significantly higher levels of posttraumatic stress symptoms (Barel, Van IJzendoorn, Sagi-Schwartz, & Bakermans-Kranenburg, 2010). At least part of what may fuel such posttraumatic stress in survivors pertains to lasting feelings of anger and hostility (Amir & Lev-Wiesel, 2003). Other studies have shown that survivors have used a variety of coping strategies that may have blends of both positive and negative emotions such as feelings of sadness, loss, and haunting memories but also trying to focus on the positive qualities of life (Mazor, Gampel, Enright, & Orenstein, 1990) and trying to detach oneself from the past trauma while also having a full realization of it (Ayalon, Perry, Arean, & Horowitz, 2007). However, it is generally believed that survivors have largely tried—and have found some success—in trying to make sense of their trauma by fundamentally focusing on beliefs and actions that are prosocial to themselves, their families, and the larger society (Armour, 2010).

In considering the meaning of the Holocaust, while survivors have naturally been emphasized, even amongst this group, there can be unique challenges faced by survivors depending on the specific circumstances related to their experience, such as whether one was a hidden child of the Holocaust (Fossion et al., 2014). Considerable attention has also been given to how survivors may transmit their experiences of Holocaust-related trauma to their offspring in both conscious and unconscious ways such that survivors and their offspring often have to work to understand and cope with the trauma that occurred to them and their lives which is also infused with their family and religious and cultural identity (e.g., Bar-On, 1998). More recent research has shown that such trauma may even be transmitted via biogenetic pathways that are, in part, influenced through epigenetic influences that change gene expression (e.g., Bowers & Yehuda, 2016); for instance, compared with controls, the offspring of Holocaust survivors showed a different pattern of gene encoding, which, in turn, was associated with a propensity for greater psychological vulnerability (Yehuda et al., 2016). Earlier research on the impact of the Holocaust for survivors primarily focused on the possible ill effects on internalizing parental and familial trauma (Solkoff, 1981); more recent work has suggested that such traumatic family histories may actually strengthen parent–child bonds (Mazor & Tal, 1996). Although the offspring of survivors may not necessarily show overt anger toward their parents, Holocaust-related frustrations and tensions often exist in both spoken and unspoken ways (Wiseman, Metzl, & Barber, 2006). To the degree that offspring of Holocaust survivors have shown difficulties with the expression of anger, it appears to be more focused on problems with inhibition and internalization of hostile feelings rather than lashing out at others per se (Gangi, Talamo, & Ferracuti, 2009).

Zahava Solomon (1995) offers an intriguing analysis as to why both the mental health of survivors and the larger psychological impact of the Holocaust largely was left unanswered for several decades since the end of World War II. Many of those reactions centered on how survivors perceived themselves and were perceived by others. To both Jewish survivors and non-survivors, there was an initial desire to not dwell on the trauma of the Holocaust, in part, due to a concern to not portray an image that Jews showed weakness or passivity during that time. However, other subsequent events helped to reestablish the urgency of examining the impact of the Holocaust including the 1961 Eichmann trial and the 1967 and 1973 Israeli Wars. Both of these events highlighted the past traumas and triumphs of the Jewish people particularly when facing existential threats of existence. And, yet, Solomon (1995) concludes her analysis with some degree of sorrow:

> It seems that the fragmentation that exists in the scientific literature on this subject is yet another manifestation of the ambivalence and even denial of the trauma victims suffering and the universal human tendency of avoidance and alienation that survivors repeatedly experience. (p. 227)

Some of the challenges in understanding the larger meaning of the Holocaust become increasingly complex when seeking to understand its larger contemporary significance to society today, with particular attention to its significance to Jews today (E. D. Miller, 2014). The late historian Peter Novick (1999) argued in *The Holocaust in American Life* that American Jews, in particular, place too much emphasis on the Holocaust. He suggests that this is regrettable in two basic respects: First, it causes Jews to dwell too much on the negativity of the Holocaust as a central form of identity and also it does not really serve as an appropriate means for reflection insomuch that the Holocaust as an event was the result of a very unique combination of factors that produced this genocide. However, a 2013 Pew research survey (Pew Research Center, 2013) of American Jews found the single-most essential part of being Jewish was "remembering the Holocaust." Furthermore, Vollhardt (2013) found experimental evidence for greater prosocial responses from Jewish participants in regards to outgroup victims when Holocaust-related themes were salient. Much greater research is needed to ascertain how larger populations may perceive or understand the Holocaust to be relevant today in both a general and personal sense. Likewise, much greater attention is needed with respect to how (if at all) Jews incorporate the Holocaust into their self-identity.

## Conclusion

The Holocaust remains one of the most difficult yet important areas to study. Although psychology has and should continue to offer perspective into how one of history's worst acts were able to be committed, the field of psychology can only offer limited insight insomuch that, as a historical and exceptionally complex event featuring grotesque violence, the study of the Holocaust may perhaps be best understood with an interdisciplinary perspective. Of course, we cannot go back in time and study precisely how individuals reacted to Hitler. Although we can, as one experiment did, ask whether individuals would personally kill Hitler if they could (Friesdorf, Conway, & Gawronski, 2015). More to the point, although we can ask individuals to categorize evil and senseless violence—particularly in the context of the Holocaust—individuals will invariably disagree as how to do so. For instance, when U.S. President Barack Obama lamented about the "senseless violence" of the Holocaust, a commentator from a conservative publication took issue with the term "senseless" given that the Nazis knew what they were doing (Johnson, 2013). Perhaps though this criticism could be considered from two equally reasonable views: That is, while there was a sensible logic to the Holocaust (from the perspective of Nazis and their sympathizers), when we consider the total brutality of the Holocaust today, the violence that ensued truly in so many ways remains profoundly challenging to comprehend today. We do know that the Holocaust still to this day has had a devastating impact on the worldwide Jewish population: Demographic estimates suggest that the worldwide Jewish population today could be twice as large if the Holocaust never occurred (Ilany, 2009). However, some counterfactual analyses of history have suggested that perhaps had the Holocaust had never occurred, American Jews (at least) may not have enjoyed as fruitful an existence as they do today; though such analyses are inherently speculative, it has been argued that the Holocaust fostered a sense of empowerment and activism in American Jews (which was the largest cohort of Jews in the world immediately following the Holocaust)—both within American society itself and support for Israel and Jewish causes—that might not have necessarily happened without the occurrence of the Holocaust (Ghert-Zand, 2015).

Perhaps what is so haunting—and horrific—to consider is what actually occurred to Jews during the Holocaust and the degree to which it occurred. At some level, suffering is suffering. Whether we consider America's troubled history of slavery, Jim Crow laws, and lynchings to terroristic or other (seemingly) random acts of violence, we cannot downplay such acts of suffering. Yet, the Holocaust clearly shows that individuals truly are capable of committing wanton acts of violence on a large, devious scale without any regard for the particulars of the victims as individuals. In that respect, it is also troubling that popular media culture often seeks to portray "Nazi Zombies" perhaps as a way to face previous and current anxieties (e.g., Webley, 2015). Such depictions likely serve to depict Nazis as monstrous boogeymen rather than seemingly 'normal' individuals who have had either ignored, grew indifferent, or encouraged violence, hatred, and genocide during the Nazi era; moreover, such images might allow us to erroneously conclude that individuals today are incapable of showing similar destructive behaviors under certain circumstances.

Another critical aspect of this article involved a consideration of the publicly available photographs and videos that have documented the destruction of the Holocaust with particular emphasis on their ever-greater prevalence on the Internet. This article has highlighted some of the potential benefits and challenges of this reality. If nothing else, these images allow us to remember that those who died in the Holocaust really did have vibrant lives and it also forces us to try to comprehend that they died under some of the most unimaginable conditions possible. If we examine these images, what might seem unimaginable can at least be somewhat better understood.

## References

Amir, M., & Lev-Wiesel, R. (2003). Time does not heal all wounds: Quality of life and psychological distress of people who survived the Holocaust as children 55 years later. *Journal of Traumatic Stress, 16*, 295–299.

Arendt, H. (1963). *Eichmann in Jerusalem: A report on the banality of evil.* New York, NY: Viking.

Armour, M. (2010). Meaning making in survivorship: Application to Holocaust survivors. *Journal of Human Behavior in the Social Environment, 20*, 440–468. doi.org/10.1080/10911350903274997

Ayalon, L., Perry, C., Arean, P. A., & Horowitz, M. J. (2007). Making sense of the past—Perspectives on resilience among Holocaust survivors. *Journal of Loss and Trauma, 12*, 281–293. doi.org/10.1080/15325020701274726

Bar-On, D. (1998) *Fear and hope: Three generations of the Holocaust*. Cambridge, MA: Harvard University Press.

Barel, E., Van IJzendoorn, M. H., Sagi-Schwartz, A., & Bakermans-Kranenburg, M. J. (2010). Surviving the Holocaust: A meta-analysis of the long-term sequelae of a genocide. *Psychological Bulletin, 136*, 677–698. doi.org/10.1037/a0020339.

Baumeister, R. F. (1999). *Evil: Inside human violence and cruelty*. New York, NY: Holt.

Beir, R. L., & Josepher, B. (2013). *Roosevelt and the Holocaust: How FDR saved the Jews and brought hope to a nation*. New York, NY: Skyhorse.

Benlolo, A. (2012, April 19). Could the Internet have stopped the Holocaust?. *The Huffington Post*. Retrieved from http://www.huffingtonpost.ca/avi-benlolo/could-the-internet-have-s_b_1434358.html

Berkowitz, L. (1999). Evil is more than banal: Situationism and the concept of evil. *Personality and Social Psychology Review, 3*, 246–253. doi.org/10.1207/s15327957pspr0303_7

Blass, T. (1998). The roots of Stanley Milgram's obedience experiments and their relevance to the Holocaust. *Analyse & Kritik, 20*, 46–53.

Bowers, M. E., & Yehuda, R. (2016). Intergenerational transmission of stress in humans. *Neuropsychopharmacology, 41*, 232–244. doi.org/10.1038/npp.2015.247

Bronner, S. E. (1999). Making sense of Hell: Three meditations on the Holocaust. *Political Studies, 47*, 314–328.

Campbell, D. (2004). Horrific blindness: Images of death in contemporary media. *Journal for Cultural Research, 8*, 55–74. doi.org/10.1080/1479758042000196971

Darley, J. M. (1999). Methods for the study of evil-doing actions. *Personality and Social Psychology Review, 3*, 269–275. doi.org/10.1207/s15327957pspr0303_9

Davies, J. (2007). Display, identity and the everyday: Self-presentation through online image sharing. *Discourse: Studies in the Cultural Politics of Education, 28*, 549–564. doi.org/10.1080/01596300701625305

Donadio, R. (2015, May 21). At Cannes, director of Holocaust film criticizes conventional approach of 'Schindler's List'. *The New York Times*. Retrieved from http://artsbeat.blogs.nytimes.com/2015/05/21/at-cannes-director-of-holocaust-film-criticizes-conventional-approach-of-schindlers-list/

Duck, W. (2009). "Senseless" violence Making sense of murder. *Ethnography, 10*, 417–434.

Fettweis, C. J. (2003). War as catalyst: moving World War II to the center of Holocaust scholarship. *Journal of Genocide Research, 5*, 225–236.

Flanzbaum, H. (1999). The Americanization of the Holocaust. *Journal of Genocide Research, 1*, 91–104. http://dx.doi.org/10.1080/14623529908413937

Fossion, P., Leys, C., Kempenaers, C., Braun, S., Verbanck, P., & Linkowski, P. (2014). Psychological and socio-demographic data contributing to the resilience of Holocaust Survivors. *The Journal of Psychology: Interdisciplinary and Applied, 148*, 641–657. doi.org/10.1080/00223980.2013.819793

Frankl, V. E. (1959). *Man's search for meaning*. New York: Washington Square Press.

Friedrichs, D. O. (2000). The crime of the century? The case for the Holocaust. *Crime, Law and Social Change, 1*, 21–41. http://dx.doi.org/10.1023/A:1008322402290

Friesdorf, R., Conway, P., & Gawronski, B. (2015). Gender differences in responses to moral dilemmas: A process dissociation analysis. *Personality and Social Psychology Bulletin, 41*, 696–713. doi.org/10.1177/0146167215575731

Gangi, S., Talamo, A., & Ferracuti, S. (2009). The long-term effects of extreme war-related trauma on the second generation of Holocaust survivors. *Violence and Victims, 24*, 687–700. doi.org/10.1891/0886-6708.24.5.687

Ghert-Zand, R. (2015, June 2). What if the Holocaust had never happened?. *The Times of Israel*. Retrieved from http://www.timesofisrael.com/what-if-the-holocaust-had-never-happened/

Hale, M. (2015, January 25). Recalling a film from the liberation of the Camps. *The New York Times*. Retrieved from http://www.nytimes.com/2015/01/26/arts/television/night-will-fall-examines-the-making-of-a-1945-holocaust-documentary.html?smprod=nytcore-iphone

Harran, M., Kuntz, D., Lemmons, R., Michael, R. A., Pickus, K., Roth, J. K., & Edelheit, A. (2000). *The Holocaust chronicle*. Lincolnwood, IL: Publications International.

Hamill, S. D. (2016, April 25). Holocaust project focuses on what Americans knew and when. *Pittsburgh Post-Gazette*. Retrieved from http://www.post-gazette.com/local/region/2016/04/25/Holocaust-project-focuses-on-what-Americans-knew-and-when/stories/201604220173

Haslam, S. A., & Reicher, S. (2007). Beyond the banality of evil: Three dynamics of an interactionist social psychology of tyranny. *Personality and Social Psychology Bulletin, 33*, 615–622. http://dx.doi.org/10.1177/0146167206298570

Heinsohn, G. (2000). What makes the Holocaust a uniquely unique genocide?. *Journal of Genocide Research, 2*, 411–430. http://dx.doi.org/10.1080/713677615

Holocaust-era archive uploads thousands of documents. (2015, July 10). *Deutsche Welle*. Retrieved from http://www.dw.com/en/holocaust-era-archive-uploads-thousands-of-documents/a-18767042

Ilany, O. (2009, April 19). How many Jews would there be if not for the Holocaust?. *Haaretz*. Retrieved from http://www.haaretz.com/how-many-jews-would-there-be-if-not-for-the-holocaust-1.274315

Johnson, E. (2013, January 28). President Obama commemorates the 'Senseless' Holocaust. *National Review*. Retrieved from http://www.nationalreview.com/corner/339003/president-obama-commemorates-senseless-holocaust-eliana-johnson

Kershaw, I. (2005, January 23). Hitler kept himself aloof from the dirtiest work. *The Telegraph*. Retrieved from http://www.telegraph.co.uk/news/uknews/1481809/Hitler-kept-himself-aloof-from-the-dirtiest-work.html#ifrndnloc

Klarsfeld, S. (1985). *The children of Izieu: A human tragedy*. New York, NY: Harry N Abrams.

Kurtz, G. (2014). *Three minutes in Poland: Discovering a lost world in a 1938 family film*. New York, NY: Farrar, Strauss, and Giroux.

Langer, L. L. (1991). *Holocaust testimonies: The ruins of memory*. New Haven, CT: Yale University Press.

Leff, L. (2005). *Buried by the Times: The Holocaust and America's most important newspaper*. New York, NY: Cambridge, UK: Cambridge University Press.

Lerner, M. J. (1980). *The belief in a just world: A fundamental delusion*. New York, NY: Plenum Press.

Lichtblau, E. (2013, March 1). The Holocaust just got more shocking. *The New York Times*. Retrieved from http://www.nytimes.com/2013/03/03/sunday-review/the-holocaust-just-got-more-shocking.html

Lodewijkx, H. F., Wildschut, T., Nijstad, B. A., Savenije, W., & Smit, M. (2001). In a violent world a just world makes sense: The case of "senseless violence" in The Netherlands. *Social Justice Research, 14*, 79–94.

Łysak, T. (2016). The posthumous life of Nazi Propaganda: Postwar films on the Warsaw Ghetto. *Apparatus: Film, Media and Digital Cultures in Central and Eastern Europe, 2*, 1–16. doi.org/10.17892/app.2016.0002.17

Mazor, A., Gampel, Y., Enright, R. D., & Orenstein, R. (1990). Holocaust survivors: Coping with post-–traumatic memories in childhood and 40 years later. *Journal of Traumatic Stress, 3*, 1–14.

Mazor, A., & Tal, I. (1996). Intergenerational transmission: The individuation process and the capacity for intimacy of adult children of Holocaust survivors. *Contemporary Family Therapy, 18*, 95–113.

McMillan, D. (2014). *How could this happen: Explaining the Holocaust*. New York, NY: Basic Books.

Miller, A. G. (2014). The explanatory value of Milgram's obedience experiments: A contemporary appraisal. *Journal of Social Issues, 70*, 558–573. doi.org/10.1111/josi.12078

Miller, E. D. (2011). Finding meaning at Ground Zero for future generations: Some reflections one decade after 9/11. *International Social Science Review, 86*, 113–133.

Miller, E. D. (2014). The double-edged sword of remembering the Holocaust: The case of Jewish self-identity. In V. Khiterer, R. Barrick, & D. Misal (Eds.), *The Holocaust: Memories and history* (pp. 133–142). Newcastle upon Tyne, UK: Cambridge Scholars Publishing.

Miller, E. D. (2015). Content analysis of select YouTube postings: Comparisons of reactions to the Sandy Hook and Aurora Shootings and Hurricane Sandy. *Cyberpsychology, Behavior, and Social Networking, 18*, 635–640. doi.org/10.1089/cyber.2015.0045

Milgram, S. (1963). Behavioral study of obedience. *Journal of Abnormal and Social Psychology, 67*, 371–378.

Milgram, S. (1974). *Obedience to authority: An experimental view*. New York, NY: Harper & Row.

Moor, P. J., Heuvelman, A., & Verleur, R. (2010). Flaming on Youtube. *Computers in Human Behavior, 26*, 1536–1546, doi.org/10.1016/j.chb.2010.05.023

Moshman, D. (2001). Conceptual constraints on thinking about genocide. *Journal of Genocide Research, 3*, 431–450. doi.org/10.1080/14623520120097224

Novick, P. (1999). *The Holocaust in American life*. New York, NY: Houghton Mifflin.

Opotow, S. (2011). How this was possible: Interpreting the Holocaust. *Journal of Social Issues, 67*, 205–224. doi.org/10.1111/j.1540-4560.2010.01694.x

Orbán, K. (2007). Trauma and visuality: Art Spiegelman's *Maus* and *In the Shadow of No Towers*. *Representations, 97*, 57–80. doi.org/10.1525/rep.2007.97.1.57

Pavlát, L. (2008). The Jewish Museum in Prague during the Second World War. *European Judaism: A Journal for the New Europe, 41*, 124–130.

Peralta, E. (2014, August 29). U.N.: Syrian refugee crisis Is 'biggest humanitarian emergency of our era'. *NPR*. Retrieved from http://www.npr.org/sections/thetwo-way/2014/08/29/344219323/u-n-syrian-refugee-crisis-is-biggest-humanitarian-emergency-of-our-era

Pew Research Center. (2013, October 1). Chapter 3: Jewish identity. *Pew Research Center: Religion & Public Life*. Retrieved from http://www.pewforum.org/2013/10/01/chapter-3-jewish-identity/

Rassin, E., Rootselaar, A. F., Heiden, S., Ugahary, A., & Wagener, S. (2005). Nazi cruelties: Are they literally hard to imagine?. *British Journal of Psychology, 96*, 321–330. doi.org/10.1348/000712605X48980

Reicher, S. D., Haslam, S. A., & Miller, A. G. (2014). What makes a person a perpetrator? The intellectual, moral, and methodological arguments for revisiting Milgram's research on the influence of authority. *Journal of Social Issues, 70*, 393–408. doi.org/10.1111/josi.12067

Schabas, W. A. (2000). Problems of international codification—Were the atrocities in Cambodia and Kosovo Genocide?. *New England Law Review, 34*, 287–302.

Solkoff, N. (1981). Children of survivors of the Nazi Holocaust: A critical review of the literature. *American Journal of Orthopsychiatry, 51*, 29–42. doi.org/10.1111/j.1939-0025.1981.tb01345.x

Solomon, Z. (1995). From denial to recognition: Attitudes toward Holocaust survivors from World War II to the present. *Journal of Traumatic Stress, 8*, 215–228. doi.org/10.1002/jts.2490080203

Staub, E. (1989). *The roots of evil: The origins of genocide and other group violence*. New York, NY: Cambridge University Press.

Staub, E. (1999). The roots of evil: Social conditions, culture, personality, and basic human needs. *Personality and Social Psychology Review, 3*, 179–192. http://dx.doi.org/10.1207/s15327957pspr0303_2

Staub, E. (2014). Obeying, joining, following, resisting, and other processes in the Milgram studies, and in the Holocaust and other genocides: Situations, personality, and bystanders. *Journal of Social Issues, 70*, 501–514. http://dx.doi.org/10.1111/josi.12074

Van Zomeren, M., & Lodewijkx, H. F. (2005). Motivated responses to "senseless" violence: Explaining emotional and behavioural responses through person and position identification. *European Journal of Social Psychology, 35*, 755–766. http://dx.doi.org/10.1002/ejsp.274

Vollhardt, J. R. (2013). "Crime against Humanity" or "Crime against Jews"? Acknowledgment in construals of the Holocaust and its importance for intergroup relations. *Journal of Social Issues, 69*, 144–161. doi.org/10.1111/josi.12008

Webley, S. (2015). The supernatural, Nazi zombies, and the play instinct: The gamification of war and the reality of the military industrial complex. In C. J. Miller & A. Bowdoin Van Riper (Eds.), *Horrors of War: The Undead on the Battlefield* (pp. 201–217). Lanham, MD: Rowman & Littlefield.

Welner, M. (2009). The justice and therapeutic promise of science-based research on criminal evil. *The Journal of the American Academy of Psychiatry and the Law, 4*, 442–449.

Wiesel, E. (1958/2006). *Night*. New York, NY: Farrar, Strauss and Giroux.

Wiseman, H., Metzl, E., & Barber, J. P. (2006). Anger, guilt, and intergenerational communication of trauma in the interpersonal narratives of second generation Holocaust survivors. *American Journal of Orthopsychiatry, 76*, 176–184. doi.org/10.1037/0002-9432.76.2.176

Wohl, M. J. A., & Van Bavel, J. J. (2011). Is identifying with a historically victimized group good or bad for your health? Transgenerational post-traumatic stress and collective victimization. *European Journal of Social Psychology, 41*, 818–824. doi.org/10.1002/ejsp.844

Wyman, D. S. (1984). *The Abandonment of the Jews: America and the Holocaust*. New York, NY: Pantheon Books.

Yehuda, R., Daskalakis, N. P., Bierer, L. M., Bader, H. N., Klengel, T., Holsboer, F., & Binder, E. B. (2016). Holocaust exposure induced intergenerational effects on FKBP5 methylation. *Biological Psychiatry, 80*, 372–380. doi.org/10.1016/j.biopsych.2015.08.005

Zeitz, J. (2015, November 22). Yes, it's fair to compare the plight of the Syrians to the plight of the Jews. Here's why. *Politico.* Retrieved from http://www.politico.com/magazine/story/2015/11/syrian-refugees-jews-holocaust-world-war-ii-213384

Zimbardo, P. G. (2004). A situationist perspective on the psychology of evil: Understanding how good people are transformed into perpetrators. In A. G. Miller (Ed.), *The social psychology of good and evil* (pp. 21–50). New York, NY: Guilford Press.

# Senseless Violence: An Overview

Ami Rokach

**ABSTRACT**

In this epilogue I review some of the existing literature on senseless violence, highlighting the phenomenon, examining the factors that cause people to commit such horrific deeds, and the complex thoughts, feelings, and acts that precede such senseless violence. The article ends with some reflections on what we should do as a profession and as a society to help curb this life shattering violence.

At 6:39 p.m. on Monday, February 12, 2007, 18-year-old Sulejman Talovic opened fire at the Trolley Square Mall in Salt Lake City, Utah. In a shooting spree that lasted a brief six minutes, Talovic killed five innocent people and injured four more before being shot and killed by Salt Lake City Police. According to his employer and family, earlier that day Talovic showed no signs of what was to come, working a normal eight-hour shift at Aramark Uniform Services from 9 to 5.... Because Talovic left no suicide or explanatory note, and because there is no known link between the killer and the victims, no known link between the killer and the location, no known link between any of the victims, and nothing unique about that day and that setting, the search for a motive is a more complicated and theoretical task. Sadly, the uncertainty of Talovic's motive is not unique to his case; most acts of violent public mass murder appear nonsensical or driven by distinct situational motivators. As there is no clear cut and universal cause, over the past forty years numerous factors have been offered to account for these types of shootings, including bullying, peer relations, family problems, cultural conflict, demographic change, mental illness, gun culture, copycatting, and the media. While there appears to be an element of truth in each of these perspectives, all of these isolated factors focus upon only one or two surface-level influences, thus ignoring the possibility that multiple and distinct causes are interacting with one another (VanGeem, 2010, pp. 1–2).

Thompson (2014) suggested that previously unknown places such as Pearl, Mississippi (1997); West Paducah, Kentucky (1997); Jonesboro, Arkansas (1998); Springfield, Oregon (1998); Littleton, Colorado (1999); Santee, California (2001); Red Lake, Minnesota (2005); and Chardon, Ohio (2012) have become a part of the American consciousness.

The aforementioned list reviews mass killings in the United States up until recently. However, it is clear that such horrendous events do not happen just there. Enough if we mention ISIS and beheadings, Israeli-Palestinians conflict marred by suicide bombings, parents killing their children as is happening all over the world for a variety of reasons, and numerous violent events which may not even be reported in the media. Not only that violence is not socially, culturally, and religiously condoned, but as curious creatures we make efforts to understand and learn how to deal with and hopefully prevent it from repeatedly occurring.

Aitken, Oosthuizen, Emsley, & Seedat (2008) observed that the term "mass murder" is largely defined as the killing of several victims (often numbered between three and five) in a single event. They added that unlike serial murder, which involves killing several victims over a period of time, mass murderers are commonly found to be suicidal as well as homicidal so they rarely survive the massacre. Aitken et al. (2008) explored the reasons that people commit mass murder, or for that matter simply engaged in senseless violence. These are multifaceted, spanning biological, psychological, and social factors. Biological factors may include brain pathology or psychiatric illnesses such as depression, psychosis, or personality disorders. Socially, mass murderers are isolated, lonely and bereft of intimate relations.

People commonly associate mass murder with the United States, however it is found in many countries throughout the world. For example, 14 of the deadly school attacks that have occurred in the last decade or so span eight different countries, six in America, two in China, and one each in Canada, Britain, Japan, Yemen, Germany, and Finland (Aitken et al., 2008).

### Factors Common to Mass Murderers

The most salient feelings that were identified by mass murderers were anger, revenge, and social alienation. These perpetrators were almost always the subject of bullying in childhood, becoming loners who felt helpless and hopeless to change their lot in life. "They were suspicious, resentful, grudge holders, who demonstrated obsessional or rigid traits. Narcissistic and grandiose traits were present, along with the heavy use of externalization as a way of coping. They held a worldview of others being rejecting and uncaring. As a result, they spent a great deal of time feeling resentful, and ruminating on past humiliations. These ruminations invariably evolved into fantasies of violent revenge. Offenders seemed to "welcome death," even perceiving it as bringing them fame with an aura of power" (Knoll 2012; p. 758). Additionally, mass murders were observed to suffer from depression, psychosis, and/or personality disorder. They were people who suffered from bullying in their childhood and adults and felt alienated and even rejected by society and by those around them (Knoll, 2012).

In the past, theories that attempted to define and explain mass murderers were mostly concerned with categorization of the crime based upon an unfocused (and often poorly delineated) collection of factors, inconsistently combining motivation, methods, and any pre-existing relationship between the offender and his victims. However, in 1986 Dietz published his theoretical categorization of mass murderers. He distinguished between family annihilators (those that target family members, usually in a home setting); those he termed "pseudocommandos" that were composed of military types dressed in fatigues and who seemed fascinated with assault weapons and symbols of power, and the set-and-run killers such as the murderers known to utilize poison or bombs in order to cause remote murders that they can escape from or not be incriminated for. In the 1990s many criminologists found these typologies to be too inconsistent and decided the scope of emphasis should be targeted squarely at motivation alone (Fox & Levin 1998).

Utilizing this new focus, crime theorists identified several categories of motivation. For instance, Fox and Levin (1998) cited vengeance related to paranoia and hostility, regarding society at large, as the most common causes. They also identified motives based upon a warped sense of love which were specifically identified in those involved in family massacres, murderers oriented toward profit which could be either monetary or political, such as acts of terrorism, and crimes motivated by a skewed thirst for individual power (popular among pseudocommandos). Kelleher (1997) developed a seven-category typology of motivation that included "most of these categories above with the addition of insanity-driven mass homicide, sexual homicide and —perverted love, a motivator typical of serial murderers" (p. 5). As senseless violence is becoming more frequent and disturbing, there are more attempts to understand what, why, and who does those horrific acts.

VanGeem (2010) reviewed the characteristics of the perpetrators of senseless violence. He asserted that they are found within three instances: (1) *Social Capital*, which is the little access that the shooter has to status and connections in the community; (2) His interpretation of that marginalization as a form of unending *victimization*; and (3) the perception of himself as a *pariah* that he adopts and resents. We know that many people feel marginalized within their everyday social circles, and others suffer from psychological impairments that negatively affect their common social interactions, but the potential shooter's self-perception is what separates him out as unique. Eventually, increased aggression and then violence become the only way he knows and can express his turmoil, and when there is a trigger, he explodes and shoots to kill those unfortunates who are at the wrong place in the wrong time (Katz, 1988).

### Social Capital

Social exchange is pursued in order to gain something desired. Usually, argues VanGeem, what is sought is dominance, as everyone wants to be in a higher position socially, than he is. This drive is tied to mechanisms of social exchange, status, prestige and reputation maintenance, hierarchy negotiation, and aggression (see also Simmel, 1950). Research indicated that senseless violence is overwhelmingly perpetrated by lonely or rejected and marginalized young males, especially unmarried ones (Hudson & den Boer, 2002; Mesquida & Wiener, 1996), who are found to be more competitive, more aggressive, and more likely to kill and be killed (Andersson, 1994).

### The Impaired Psyche

Newman (2004) indicated that at least 52% of those who committed senseless violence suffered from a serious mental illness, such as schizophrenia or a bipolar disorder at the time of the shooting. He added that personal psychologies, whether classified in the DSM or not, are important as they magnify the social marginalization and alienation. For instance, Sampson and Laub (1993) argued that social bonds are more malleable and situation specific. And so, impulsive risk-taking is a more appealing line of action when social bonds between a delinquent and the larger society are weak. "Although background factors such as structural disadvantage and chaotic familial relations can significantly compromise social bonds in childhood and negatively affect youth delinquency and deviance, in adulthood, positive marriage attachment and job attachment serve as mechanisms of change"(VanGeem, 2010; p. 21).

### The Pariah Self-Image

Senseless violence is perpetrated by mostly males whose main characteristic is self-loathing. Thus, a random, senseless murder allows the offender to cement a new, more thrilling self-image, and to prove that he can break whatever rules he wants. In order for, what Katz (1988) termed, the "bad ass" to set himself apart from all those who are not real bad asses, tough and worthwhile, he needs to show that he is not kidding, and unlike the pretenders, his retribution will be swift, certain, and merciless. That, in his eyes, qualifies him to get others' respect and deference. These public shooters, as we so well know, are not seeking anonymity. On the contrary, in the majority of cases they go as far as to advertise their impending crimes to multiple people beforehand. The public stage is set and the pariah has openly committed him or herself to delivering a deliberate and powerful message in the only way left—violent and swift (Vossekuil, Fein, Reddy, Borum, & Modzeleski, 2002). Fox and Levin (1998) viewed the long simmering frustration and overwhelming sense of failure that pushes the individual towards such violence. They identified such feelings as self-hate, worthlessness, and blaming one's own weakness for the undesirable situation he finds himself in. That could lead to suicide and or physical harm to oneself. However, when the individual perceives himself as victim, as a pariah who loathes his position in society, the aggression is directed outwards and adopting a moral righteousness, external aggression facilitates justification for the slaughter that follows. As VanGeem (2010) summarized it "an individual suffering from low social status, filtered through the skewed lens of psychological impairment, —rationally‖ develops a pariah self-image fixated upon a violent solution. In that situation, the individual is only looking for the most appropriate way to effectively cause chaos, fear, and pain; he or she relies upon —cultural scripts geared toward this end" (pp. 36–37).

> On Friday, December 14, 2012, a deranged 20-year-old walked into Sandy Hook Elementary in Newtown, Connecticut, and executed 20 young children and six teachers and administrators. …The statistics are frightening. Between 1997 and 2012, ten boys have killed 73 students, parents, and teachers, and wounded 99 more, in the nine most well publicized school shootings. (Thompson, 2014; p. 210).

## *Future Directions*

What can be done to curb or even prevent mass murder and other senseless violence? Research indicates several areas that we need to focus on in order to better understand how to handle such situations and destructive events. It is important to know what *victim characteristics* are. Senseless violence may be practiced on complete strangers, but more often than not, it is the fate of people who may know the perpetrators, who belong to a specific group/ religion/or culture. A *motive* may vary between crimes and among perpetrators, but there is always a motive, mostly grounded in hate and a wish to destroy. What was the *weapon* used, and is there a way for society to restrict people's access to those weapons? Palermo (2007) described mass murder as a "culmination of a continuum of experiences, perceptions, beliefs, frustrations, disappointments, hostile fantasies, and perhaps pathology" (p. 18). This may apply to various acts of senseless violence, but needs to be researched and verified.

Bowers, Holmes and Rhom (2010) observed that research has suggested that mass murderers have been frequently found to possess atypical behaviors and/or some of the cluster B personality traits, which include, among other characteristics: antisocial personality, narcissism, hostility, oversensitive, rigid with obsessional traits, self-righteous, grandiose traits (i.e., a sense of entitlement), and impulsivity. We need to develop effective ways of assessing, identifying, and attending to those individuals before—way before—they become dangerous and destructive.

## References

Aitken, L., Oosthuizen, P., Emsley, R., & Seedat, S. (2008). Mass murders: Implications for mental health professionals. *International Journal of Psychiatry in Medicine, 38*(3), 261–9.

Andersson, M. B. (1994). *Sexual selection.* Princeton, NJ: Princeton University Press.

Bowers, T. G., Holmes, E. S., & Rhom, A. (2010). The nature of mass murder and autogenic massacre. *Journal of Police and Criminal Psychology, 25*(2), 59–66.

Dietz, P. E. (1986). Mass, serial, and sensational homicides. *Bulletin of the New York Academy of Medicine,* (62), 477–491.

Fox, J. A., &. Levin, J. (1998). Multiple homicide: Patterns of serial and mass murder. *Crime and Justice,* (23), 407–455.

Hudson, V., & den Boer, A. (2002). A Surplus of Men, a Deficit of Peace: Security and Sex Ratios in Asia's Largest States. *International Security* (26), 5–38.

Katz, J. (1988). *Seductions of crime: Moral and sensual attractions in doing evil.* New York, NY: Basic Books.

Kelleher, M. D. (1997). *Flashpoint: The American mass murderer.* Westport, CT: Praeger.

Knoll, J. L., IV. (2012). Mass murder: Causes, classification, and prevention. *Psychiatric Clinics of North America, 35*(4), 757–780.

Mesquida, C., & Wiener, N. (1996). Human Collective Aggression: A Behavioral Ecology Perspective. *Ethology and Sociobiology* (17), 247–262.

Newman, K. S. (2004). *Rampage: The social roots of school shootings.* Cambridge, MA: Perseus Book Group.

Palermo, G. B. (2007). Homicidal syndromes: a clinical psychiatric perspective. In Kocsis, R. N. (ed.), *Criminal profiling: International theory, research, and practice* (pp. 3–26). Totowa, NJ: Humana Press.

Sampson, R. J., & Laub, J. H. (1993). *Crime in the Making: Pathways and turning points through life.* Cambridge, MA: Harvard University.

Simmel, G. (1950). *The Sociology of Georg Simmel,* edited by K. Wolf. Glencoe, IL: The Free Press.

Thompson, C. B. (2014). Our killing schools. *Society, 51*(3), 210–220.

VanGeem, S. (2010). Status and slaughter: The psycho-social factors that influence public mass murder. *Sociological Abstracts.* UMI Number: 1470119.

Vossekuil, B., Fein, R. A., Reddy, M., Borum, R., & Modzeleski, W. (2002). *The final report and findings of the safe school initiative: Implications for the prevention of school attacks in the United States.* Washington, DC: U.S. Secret Service National Threat Assessment Center and U.S. Department of Education.

# Index

*Note*: Boldface page numbers refer to tables.

accidental death 42
activism 11
acute psychotic filicide 42
acute strain 25
ADHD *see* attention-deficit/hyperactivity
    disorder
altruism 42–3
altruistic filicide 42
antisocial thoughts and behaviors 13–14
April 1999 Columbine massacre 24
Arendt, Hannah 89
Asperger's syndrome 58–60
atmosphere game 78
attention-deficit/hyperactivity disorder
    (ADHD) 60
autism spectrum disorders (ASDs) 3; and
    criminal behavior 49–50; mass shooters 51–4;
    mass shootings *see* mass shootings; mental
    illness 51–2; monoamine oxidase A 50–1

"banality of evil" 89
Berkowitz, Leonard 90
brutality 90

Central American: political dysfunction 70–1;
    refugee crisis 69–74
child murder 36
chronic strains 25
collateral damage 10
Columbine killers 25
Columbine mass murder 61
*Columbine Report* 30
content-based ratings 77
contextualism, developmental 10–12
cosmic connectedness 8
crime rate in U.S. 22
Criminal Autistic Psychopathy 58
cumulative strain theory 25

Day of Retribution 59
developmental contextualism 10–12
*Diary of Anne Frank, The* 92

Einsatzgruppen 90
El Salvador, refugee crisis 70
Entertainment Software Rating Board (ESRB)
    77, **80**, **81**, 80–4

Farabundo Martí National Liberation Front
    (FMLN) 70
fatal maltreatment filicide 42
feminist scholarship 11
filicidal fathers 37
FMLN *see* Farabundo Martí National
    Liberation Front

Gardner, Alexander 94
government shootings 23
gratuitous violence 6
Guatemala, refugee crisis 71
gun violence 7

Harris, Eric 25
High School Shootings 53
Hobbes, Thomas 7
Holocaust: in human history 88–9; making
    sense of 99–101; post-traumatic symptoms 98;
    senseless violence and evil 89–99
*Holocaust in American Life, The* 101
Honduras, refugee crisis 70
human geography 15

IDSA *see* Interactive Digital Software
    Association
individual perpetrators 24
Interactive Digital Software Association
    (IDSA) 77
intersectionality 11
ISIS attacks 1–2

"Jewish Life in Bialystok" 96
Jews during Holocaust 88–102

Khmer Rouge 92
Klebold, Dylan 25
Kosovo conflicts 92

macro-sociological level 24–5
maladaptive development/trajectories 14–15
*Man's Search for Meaning* (Frankl) 99
mass murder 23, 108–10
mass shooters 51–4
mass shootings 51, **55**; case study 55–8;
    challenges in conducting research 52; database
    searches 54–5; Google Scholar 55; Path to
    Intended Violence 52–3; present study 53
media, affecting sensibility of violence 8–9
mental illness 51–2
mentally abnormal offenders 50
microaggressions 14, 15
micro-social interpersonal level 24
Miller, Arthur 90
monoamine oxidase A (MAO-A) 50–1
mood disorder and depression 40–1
*Mother Jones* 27
Mother Jones mass shooter database 53–4; case
    study **55**, 55–8; limitations 61; research 61–2;
    review findings 58–60
MS-13 71
multi-axis social identities 15

National Latino Psychology Association
    (NLPA) 73
Nazi Zombies 102
Novick, Peter 101

pariah self-image 109–10
participatory action research (PAR) study 15
paternal filicide-suicide 37; altruism 42–3;
    classification of 42; method 38–9; motives
    42–3; offence 39–40; personality disorder
    43–5; post-offence pathology 41; pre-offence
    pathology 40–1; spousal revenge 42
perception-making processes 8
personality disorder 43–5
Pew research survey (2013) 101
post-offence pathology 41
pre-offence pathology 40–1
proocial thoughts and behaviors 13–14
psychological well-being 14

Radford data collection effort 61
Radford/FGCU Serial Killer Database 61–2
rampage school shootings 7; definition 21;
    deterioration, unqualified 27–8; offenders
    24–6; patternless 26–7; patternlessness 29–30;
    pervasive misperception 23; randomness

23, 28–9; risk of homicide 27–8; as social
    problem 23–4
random violence 22
*Random Violence: How We Talk about New
    Crimes and New Victims* (Best) 22
refugee crisis 69–74
Roosevelt administration 94–5

schizoaffective disorder 43
schizoid personality disorder (SPD) 43–5
school shooting 23
self-preservation 7, 15
self-sabotage 16
sense of interconnectedness 8
senseless violence 1–4; and evil 89–93; origins
    and representation of 6–7
sense-making, around violence 9–10
sensibility of violence 8–9
Serial Homicide Expertise and Information
    Sharing Collaborative (SHEISC) 61–2
social capital 109
social messages, affecting sensibility of
    violence 8–9
social problem, school rampage as 23–4
Solomon, Zahava 100–1
SPD *see* schizoid personality disorder
spousal revenge 42
spree killings 54
stratification: developmental contextualism as
    framework 10–12; psychological perspectives
    on 12–15
street fighting 71
street shootings 6
Structured Clinical Interview for DSM-IV
    Axis I and II disorders (SCID) 39
Sulzberger, Arthur 95
survivor, psychological perspective 7–8

targeted shootings 23
targeted victims, random *vs.* 27–8
terrorist attacks 1–2, 23

unaccompanied children, senseless violence
    against 69–74
uncontrolled strain 25
United States: ISIS attack 2; political response
    72; psychological and ecological implications
    and recommendations 73; refugee crisis in 69;
    undocumented, unaccompanied children to 72
unwanted filicide 42
U.S. Central Intelligence Agency 71

verstehen 22
victim, psychological perspective 7–8
victimization 109
violence: for children 14; developmental
    contextualism as framework 10–12;

internalizing 12–13; issue of deterioration 22; issue of pointlessness 22; migration of 15; psychological perspectives on 12–15; and refugee 71; rethinking sense making around 9–10; schizoid personality disorder and 44–5
violent video game (VVG): aggressive behavior 77; ESRB game-ratings 77, **80**, **81**, 80–4; massive multi-player online role-playing games 81–4; M-rated video games 78;

negative outcomes 79; rating system 78; research 80–5; third-person shooter 81; T-rated games 77, 78

Warsaw Ghetto 99
Westside Middle School massacre 61

zero tolerance environments 27
Zimbardo, Philip 91

www.ingramcontent.com/pod-product-compliance
Ingram Content Group UK Ltd.
Pitfield, Milton Keynes, MK11 3LW, UK
UKHW010021280225
455677UK00023B/729